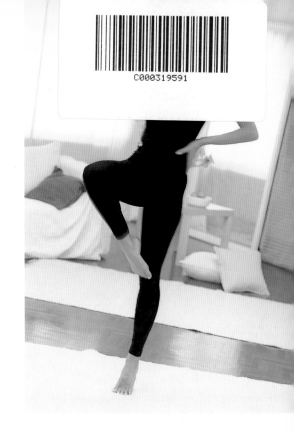

thin thighs
diet&workout

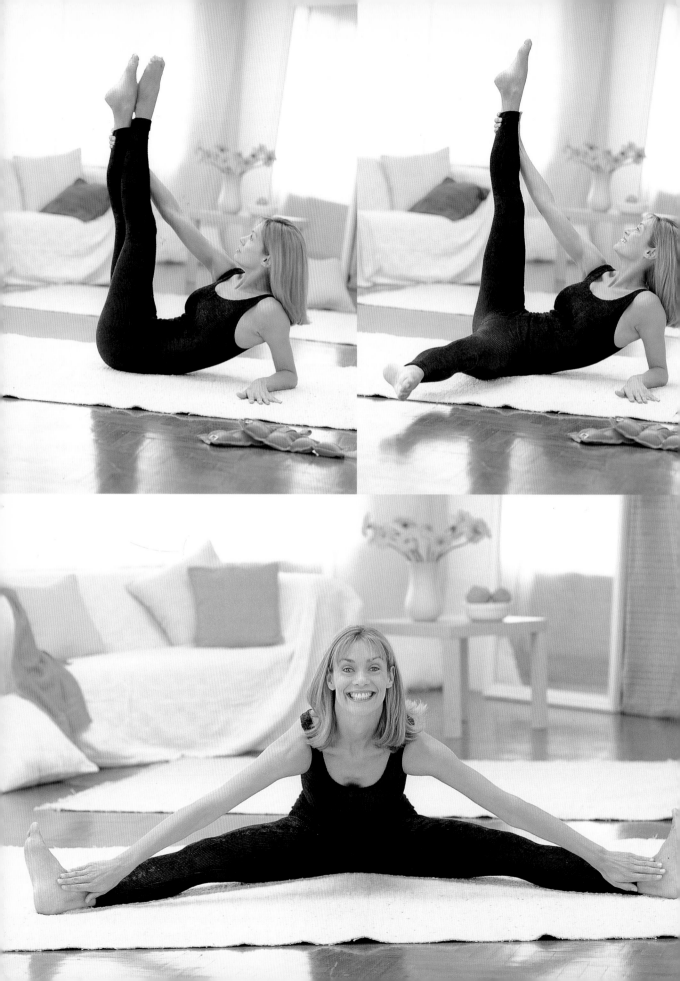

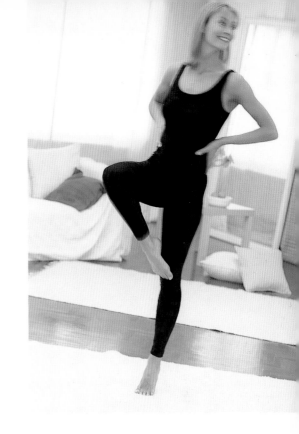

thin thighs
diet**&**workout

Karen Burke M.D., Ph.D.

hamlyn

Publishing Director: Laura Bamford
Executive Editor: Jane McIntosh
Creative Director: Keith Martin
Editors: Anne Johnson and Catharine Davey
Assistant Editor: Nicola Hodgson
Senior Designer: Louise Leffler
Designer: Paul Webbww
Mac Operator: Peter Burt
Production Controller: Julie Hadingham
Illustrator: Hilary McManus
Photographer: Peter Myers
Stylist: Elisa Palmer
Hair and Make-Up: Elinor Lindstrom and Andrea Black
Author photograph on page 4 by Manning Gurney
Insulin diagram by Paul Webb

First published in Great Britain in 1998
by Hamlyn, an imprint of Octopus Publishing Group Limited,
2–4 Heron Quays, London, E14 4JP

This edition first published 2001

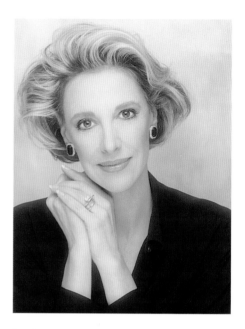

Dr. Karen Burke is a dermatologist and research scientist with a Ph.D. in biophysics from Cornell University and an M.D. from New York University. She is in private practice in New York City where she is also a Staff Member at Cabrini Medical Center.

Dr. Burke is known for her research on the prevention and reversal of aging of the skin as well as the prevention and treatment of skin cancer. She has also studied breast cancer and has published research papers on many subjects including fat structure and metabolism. She is a foremost authority in the field of cosmetic dermatology, and a frequent consultant to both pharmaceutical and cosmetic companies. Because she believes that "the best cosmetic of all is naturally healthy skin," she has researched and formulated her own exclusive line of Longévité® skin care products. Dr. Burke has written numerous articles and is frequently quoted as a health and skin care expert in magazines such as Harper's Bazaar, Glamour, Elle and Family Circle. She is the author of two successful books, Thin Thighs for Life (1995) and Great Skin for Life (1996) both published by Hamlyn, and has made numerous television and radio appearances in the USA, Great Britain, France and Germany. She lives with her husband and twin sons in New York.

Contents

Acknowledgements
With my special thanks to my husband Peter and to Heather Nolan, Dina da Silva, Arthur Burgess, Nancy Burgess, Leila Seenath, Lourdes Abrugar and Katherine Shepherd as well as to Maggie Stevens who provided the beautiful Waterford Wedgwood and Rosenthal dishes used in the recipe photographs.

A Note on Weights and Measurements
All recipes include customary metric and imperial measurements. Conversions are based on a standard developed for this book and have been rounded off. Actual weights may vary fractionally. Use only one set of measurements when preparing each recipe.

Foreword

When I wrote *Thin Thighs for Life* three years ago, I never expected such an enthusiastic response. Women from all walks of life, of all ages, from many countries, contacted me to say they were thrilled because they really lost their unattractive cellulite and improved their appearance with my plan. So many of these readers commented that they greatly enjoyed the exercises they had learned – especially as they took so little time and were very effective. They also expressed their joy in their new way of eating: they had learned how to enjoy large portions of delicious foods, and lose excess weight at the same time!

In *Thin Thighs Diet and Workout*, I will update you on new scientific advances in the regulation of hunger and in metabolism. As a physician and a scientist, I can share with you medical knowledge and techniques that will help you look more beautiful, become healthier, and be more confident and happy. I dispel misconceptions about cellulite, and tell you what it is, why it appears – and how you can reduce yours.

And in *Thin Thighs Diet and Workout*, you will learn many new ways to cook. Chapter 3 offers lots of fabulous recipes that are not only easy to prepare but also elegant enough for special guests and special occasions. You will see how to make substitutions in your own favourite recipes to make them healthy and slimming without losing their taste. You will learn to eat to nourish your body – happily and healthily, without feeling hunger or unsatisfied cravings, and to enjoy a wide variety of tastes and foods. With **GREFLOFS Great Food, Low Fat, Sugar-Free** eating, you are free to choose the foods you like. You need not follow rigid menus or buy expensive foods in speciality stores. You can eat anywhere – at home with your family or in restaurants – enjoying every meal. You won't become obsessed with a "diet". You need follow only a few simple rules, and you will learn the medical reasons for these suggestions. Knowing the "Why" will most certainly help you develop the "How"!

Thin Thighs Diet and Workout expands on the super-efficient exercise routine of *Thin Thighs for Life*, which resculpts your body and improves your posture in just twelve minutes a day. From an array of new **Thigh Thinners**, you will design your own individual intensive three-times-a-week programme. You will learn new and special **Pressometrics** that you can do any time, anywhere, to become slimmer and energized. No longer will waiting for lifts, buses or trains, sitting at your desk, at a

NOTICE

It is always advisable to check with your doctor before beginning any diet or exercise programme. If you have any medical condition for which you require a doctor's care or prescription medications or if you have had injuries which might impair exercise, be sure to discuss your diet and exercise plan with your physician before beginning. Even if you have no medical problems that you know of, this might be a good time to have a medical examination.

meeting or on the telephone, or being stuck in traffic be an exasperating waste of time!

Thin Thighs Diet and Workout updates you on the age-old custom of skin brushing and massage, using specific creams that really can help smooth that uneven, bulging cellulite. This luxury will become a part of your life – just like washing your face, and in even less time!

No matter how out of shape you may feel right now, your body can change within weeks – and starting to take control of your unwanted fat instead of allowing it to control you will make you happier and more optimistic. Your body is an amazing instrument that responds quickly to new conditioning and input. I can guarantee that if you follow the simple rules I describe, after 30 days your thighs and even your whole body will be noticeably sleeker.

You can look great and be healthy! Don't waste one more moment being self-conscious of your cellulite. Take action now! Offer yourself a wonderful lifestyle that will make you look much better and give you energy and possibly even a longer life. You deserve it! As a busy professional woman and a mother, I can promise you that you can easily incorporate this programme into your everyday life without spending a lot of time or money.

If we can make it to the moon and to Mars, we can certainly devise a pain-free system to lose a little cellulite! The strategy you are about to learn feels good, makes you happy, and is easy to incorporate into your presently active life. Let science work for you, and have fun!

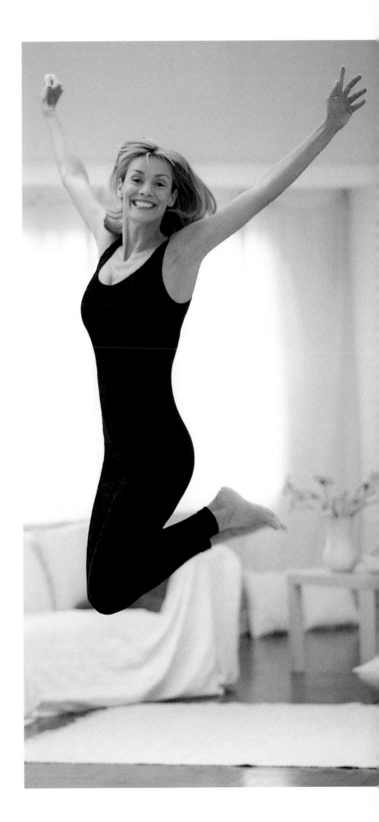

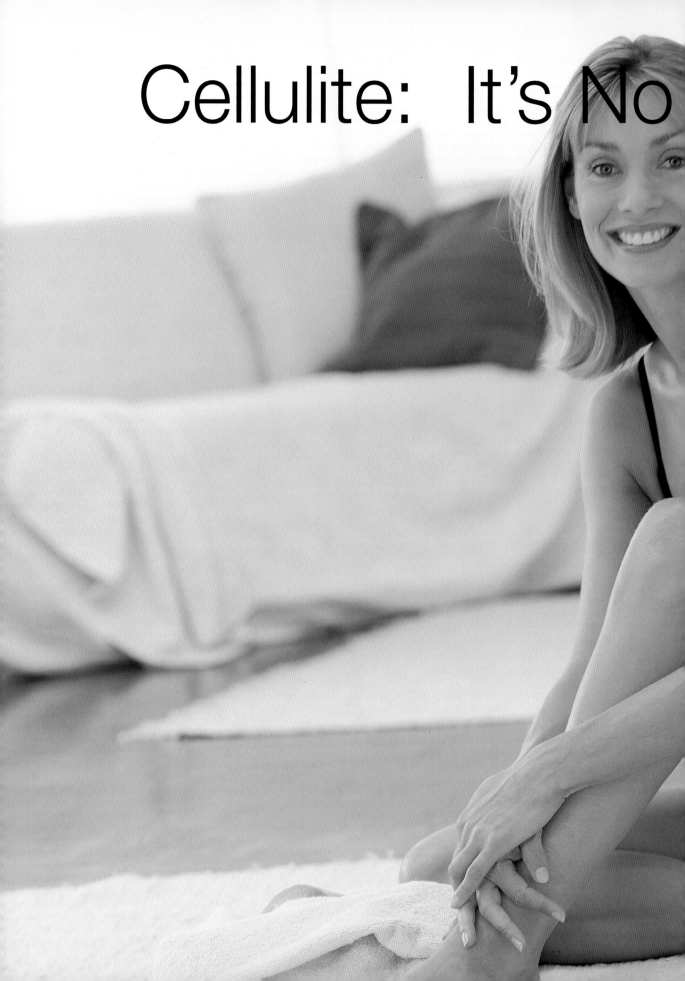

Cellulite: It's No

Mystery

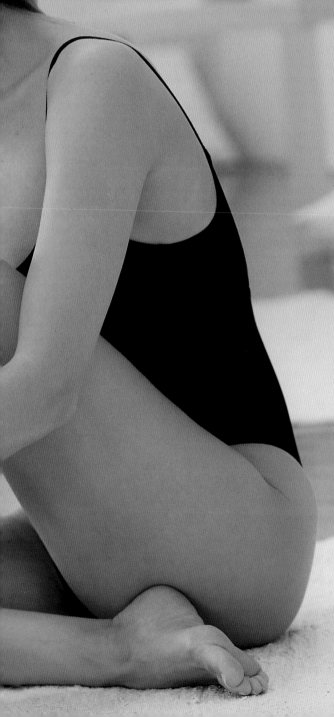

Cellulite is not a disease. It is a natural characteristic of the female body, like protruding breasts or the lack of body and facial hair. Cellulite is simply fat, but it is packaged differently in women, so where there is more fat on the female figure (especially the hips and thighs), the surface can appear dimply or lumpy.

When a young girl reaches puberty, female sexual hormones, especially oestrogen, cause her to develop breasts, hips, and the typical female curves. Oestrogen also leads to increased fat on the lower body, especially on the thighs and hips. When the female fat cells enlarge in response to increased oestrogen, the door is wide open for cellulite to appear. If and when the condition becomes noticeable, it takes on the appearance (regrettably!) of fleshy orange peel or a lumpy mattress.

Both the dimpled look and the lumpy ripples are caused by the way the fat is anchored beneath the skin and by the way this fat is stored in fat cell compartments, surrounded by thickened dividers of connective tissue. Remember, fat stored in our bodies is not firm or solid: it ripples because it is softer and more spongy in texture than our other tissue such as skin or muscle.

Sex Differences

By the late 1970s, Doctors Nuremberger and Muller in Berlin discovered a very distinct difference between the female and male structure of the connective tissue that "packages" fat cells under our skin. Following an eight-year study of the structure of female and male skin and subcutaneous fat, the doctors observed that, in women, fat cells are grouped within sacs, divided by connective tissue arranged in a vertically arched design, attached to the deep layer (the "dermis") of overlying skin to form "standing fat cell chambers". From these fat cell chambers, little anchors project upwards into the lower layer of the skin, dividing the regions of the deep dermis. As they fill with fat, these vertical fat cell chambers protrude outwards into the skin's surface. The result – the appearance of lumpy cellulite! When a sack of tomatoes is pressed tightly, the surface appears lumpy. In the same way, if fat cells inside the connective tissue sacs enlarge, as they do when you gain weight, they force the skin to stretch tightly across the fat, making your thighs look dimply.

In the comparable skin of men's thighs, the connective tissue anchors are structured in a horizontal honeycomb or lattice-like pattern, packaging fat cells in small, many-sided shapes. The connective fibres in males are not only more numerous, they also tend to penetrate at an angle, like the strings of a parachute. Because of this net-like architecture, as male fat cells enlarge, they do not protrude straight into the dermal layer of the skin, avoiding the corresponding rippling on the skin's surface. The outer layer of a man's skin is thicker than a woman's, further insulating the male from surface lumpiness. To top it all, the packages of fat in women are larger than in men (say, the size of grapes as opposed to the size of blueberries). Needless to say, a plastic bag full of grapes looks lumpier than a cloth sack full of blueberries!

This packaging of fat cells is determined by your hormones. Before birth, the male characteristics become evident only as of the sixth or seventh month, when male hormones are first formed. Only then, just before the actual birth, does the structure of the packaging of male fat cells change so that he will not develop cellulite later. Before that, his fat cell structure is just like a female's!

These differences in male and female surface and sub-surface tissue accentuate with age. As we women grow older, our connective tissue anchors thicken, while our surface skin becomes thinner and less elastic. As a result, our skin is less resistant to pressure from the bulging fat chambers beneath. More rippling can appear, and the dimpling of cellulite is more evident.

As you can see, like it or not, women are by nature susceptible to cellulite. There are differences in the texture and structure of the under-skin packaging of our fat cells, with regrettable consequences for us women!

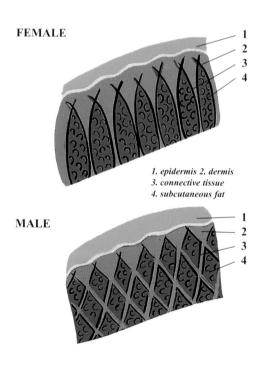

FEMALE

1
2
3
4

*1. epidermis 2. dermis
3. connective tissue
4. subcutaneous fat*

MALE

1
2
3
4

The structure of a woman's skin and connective tissue, as compared to a man's, causes the appearance of cellulite.

What about Hormones?

Hormones influence how our fat cells grow. Each of us is born with a certain number of fat cells, determined by ethnic and genetic factors. The number of our fat cells increases until the age of two, depending upon the infant's initial diet. The only other times that the number of fat cells increases are during puberty or with a major weight gain leading to obesity.

During puberty, the male hormone testosterone causes changes in connective tissue:

1 enlargement of all the muscles;

2 a decrease in the size of fat cells in the lower part of the body, the male's hips and thighs;

3 an enlargement in the size of fat cells in the shoulders and upper chest.

FEMALE

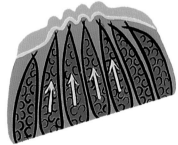

MALE

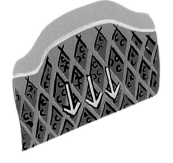

A simple "pinch test" reveals the dimpling, or orange peel effect, of cellulite on a woman's thigh, but not on a man's.

The female hormone oestrogen has a different effect:

1 no enlargement of the muscles;

2 no enlargement in the size of fat cells in the shoulders;

3 an increase in the size of fat cells below the umbilicus, particularly on the hips, buttocks and thighs. In some cases this increase may extend as far as the knees.

Furthermore, a normal woman has more fat cells than a man. In fact, an average woman of 21 has almost twice the volume of fat as does a man of the same age. Women have on average about 22 per cent body fat, while men have only 12 per cent. It's simply not fair!

Not only does oestrogen cause the localization of more and larger fat cells on the lower part of the female body, it also makes the skin's dermis layer thinner so those underlying fat cell packages are more readily seen on the surface of the skin. Men's testosterone gives the added advantage of thickening the body hair. This "buttresses" the already thicker skin, which lessens the appearance of surface rippling even further.

Finally, oestrogen causes some retention of water, unlike testosterone which does not. As a result, when female hormonal levels increase (especially during puberty or with oral contraceptives), overall water retention applies pressure, and can seem to increase cellulite.

Why Apples and Pears?

Sadly – as we know all too well – when women become overweight, their excess is concentrated on the thighs and buttocks and they become pear-shaped. Men, on the other hand, become apple-shaped, with their excess in the belly. This distribution is caused not only by hormones, but also by the enzyme on the fat cell surface responsible for transporting fat into the cell – "lipoprotein lipase". The greater the activity of this enzyme, the more fat is taken in. In women, lipoprotein lipase activity is higher in the thighs and buttocks, and in men the activity is higher in the abdomen.

Genetically heavier individuals have increased enzyme activity – as we all do when we eat sugar (since sugar causes insulin release and insulin stimulates lipoprotein lipase). With increased enzyme activity, our fat cells soak up fat like a sponge: the result, our unflattering shapes! The good news is that the activity of this lipoprotein lipase can be decreased by caffeine and certain medications. As you will learn in Chapter 5, creams with these ingredients can be massaged into the thighs to help decrease the appearance of cellulite!

What About Blood Flow?

When a woman becomes overweight, other negative factors come into play: fat cells enlarging within each sac of connective tissue cause "double trouble" – reduced blood flow and reduced drainage of the lymphatic system. Dr Sergio Curri in Milan showed that there is a fine-tuned regulation of blood flow within our fat tissue through little valves in the tiny blood vessels that supply our fat cells. If the fat cells enlarge, pressure on our micro-blood vessels causes these valves to constrict blood flow. To put it simply, when we gain weight, our circulatory system does not function to its proper standard, further contributing to the appearance of cellulite!

How is Fat Metabolized?

Our body processes ("metabolizes") fat in a chain, somewhat like a factory assembly line!

1 We absorb dietary fat from the intestines.

2 We both store and synthesize fat (as "lipid molecules") in the liver.

3 We transport this dietary fat and synthesized lipid through our bloodstream to our fat cells.

4 The enzyme lipoprotein lipase on the surface of the fat cell breaks down the fatty "triglycerides" into glycerol and free fatty acids to allow fat to enter the fat cell.

5 Triglycerides are re-formed within our fat cells for the storage of fat.

6 When we need energy, the store of triglycerides within our fat cells is again broken down and the free fatty acids are moved out to fuel our muscles.

The synthesis and storage of fats is governed by our genetics and our hormones. Certain foods and medicines can alter the process. For example, caffeine, as well as certain medicines such as theophyllin and aminophylin (which is frequently used to treat asthma), can increase the breakdown of fat. Many of the anti-cellulite creams now available on the market contain these effective compounds.

Eating foods that are too rich in fats, and eating too much (especially after a fast) activates the movement of fat into our fat cells. Lipoprotein lipase activity is increased with the release of insulin (stimulated by our eating sugar and refined carbohydrates), permitting more fat to be transported into our fat cells. Conversely, this enzyme's activity is decreased by fasting, after strenuous muscular exercise, and with lack of insulin. Need I say more? As you exercise and control your eating, you are actually reducing your body's production of the enzyme that moves fat into your fat cells!

Insulin

Our pancreas releases insulin, the hormone that regulates how our body metabolizes and stores sugar and fat. Insulin lowers blood glucose after we have eaten, directing our muscle cells and liver to store the glucose as glycogen and our liver to convert extra glucose to protein and fat. Insulin also orders our fat cells not only to take up and store fat, but also not to break down fat already stored. So to eliminate cellulite we should stop eating fat and limit insulin by avoiding sugar and insulin-releasing carbohydrates.

The Solution is Clear

All this adds up to one conclusion: cellulite is a physical fact – a reality – caused by female hormones influencing connective tissue and fat cells. As we gain weight, our fat cells enlarge within their connective tissue sacs, making our skin surface look lumpy – and constricting blood flow so our metabolism is slowed. The result is a cycle of progressively worsening cellulite! Fortunately, you will learn in Chapters 3, 4 and 5 how this cycle can be stopped!

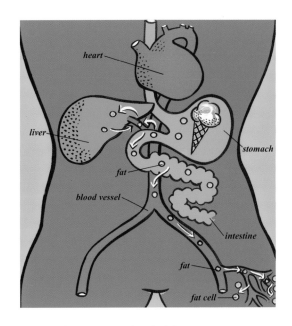

The fat you eat is absorbed from your intestine and transported through your blood, either directly or via your liver, to your fat cells.

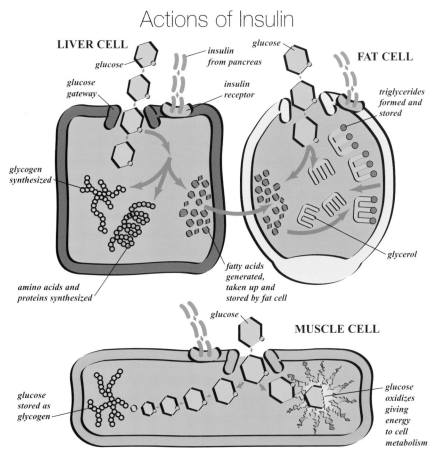

Actions of Insulin

Insulin is released when there is an increase in blood glucose after eating sugar and/or carbohydrate.

Insulin acts to ✪ increase and ✪ promote the transport of glucose into **muscle** and **fat cells**. Without insulin, these cells are impermeable to glucose, regardless of how much glucose is in the blood.

Within the fat cell, fatty acids and glycerol combine ⊕ to form triglycerides, the stored form of fat.

In **fat cells** insulin ✪ enhances the uptake of fats ⊕ promotes the storage of fat, and ⊖ inhibits the breakdown of stored fats.

In the **liver**, insulin ✪ stimulates the conversion of glucose to stored glycogen, amino acids, protein, fat and fatty acids which are used by fat cells to store even more fat.

The Cellulite-Free

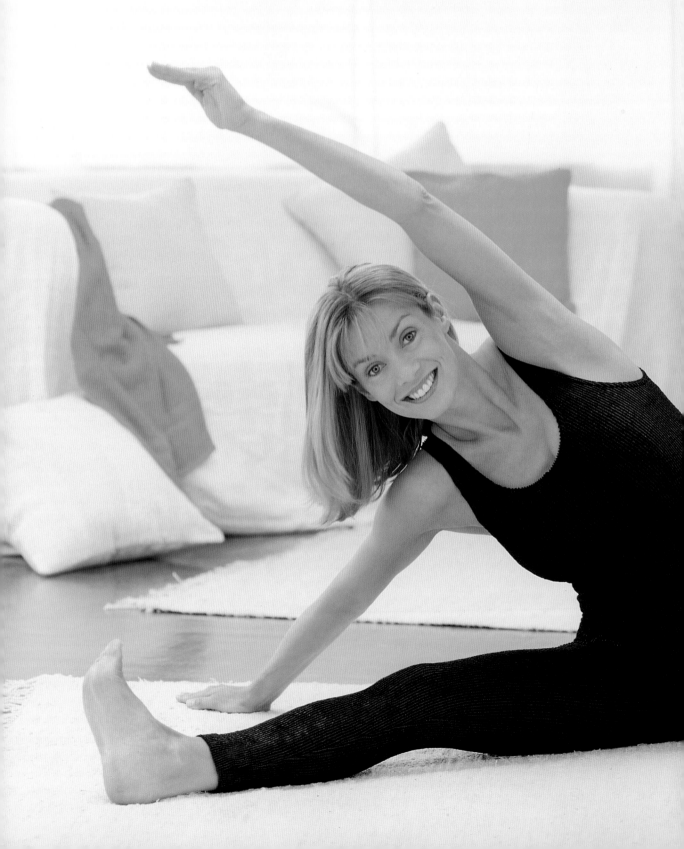

Lifestyle

You are about to learn a better, happier way of living! You will have the joy of feeling good about yourself, having more energy, and being trim, fit and cellulite-free!

You of course know the bottom line – that proper diet and exercise are the keys to your well-being and general appearance. But how do we accomplish this? We've tried in the past. What we learn in the following chapters is a lifestyle with a few easy-to-follow concepts for eating, and an incredibly efficient way to exercise in just minutes each day. This is not an unrealistic, overly-demanding plan that would yield, at best, only temporary results.

This is not like most diet and exercise programmes, which involve very complex rules, rigorous counting of calories or grams of certain nutrients, and weighing each morsel that enters your mouth. Rigid plans call for severe limitations on allowed foods, strict day-by-day menus that may not appeal to you (not to speak of your family and friends), and demanding, difficult exercise routines which are not only time consuming but also often require special equipment or facilities.

Getting Started

Instead of a complicated, rigid programme, this cellulite-free lifestyle uses concepts based on medical science that you can easily incorporate into your present routine. Certain ingredients and combinations of foods are really detrimental to your health. As you learn to avoid these, you will enjoy a great variety of new, exciting tastes. You will be introduced to some easily obtainable, new foods that are so filling that you do not want to eat some of the "extras" you automatically "shovel in". And you will learn how to eat to actually help move fat out of fat cells! There is a whole repertoire of new recipes – all so smashingly elegant that your family and guests will consider you a gourmet chef. And you will have a table of ingredient substitutions so that you can modify your favourite recipes to make them healthy, slimming and delicious.

But that's not all! There's no doubt that you can change your body's shape through exercise. And you need not be a "fitness addict" to look fantastic. The trick is to know which exercises to do! Some forms of exercise may actually increase body weight and the girth of your thighs by increasing muscle mass. Generally, muscle development can be good, but some exercises that increase muscle also make cellulite more noticeable (since the increased bulk of muscle pushes up against the overlying fat, making the skin's surface even lumpier!). The best way to decrease the appearance of cellulite is to stretch the muscles – to elongate the body. You will be presented with a unique series of exercises that really does reduce your rippling, dimpled cellulite within weeks, even as it makes you more supple and flexible. And you need not suffer to achieve your goal! The basic routine takes less than 15 minutes each day – easy to integrate into any schedule. And there's more: **Pressometrics**, exercises you can do anytime, anywhere, to thin your thighs and to give you an energy pick-up during a daytime slump; and **Thigh Thinners**, a longer, intense, fabulous exercise session.

"If there is a Why, there is always a How."
— Nietzsche

You have your own, very personal "Why": you want to look great for a specific occasion (as well as for the rest of your life); you want to feel better about yourself; you are in the mood for a positive change; you want to surprise someone special; you want more energy. Make a list of all your Whys. Stick this list by your bedside, on your make-up mirror and on your refrigerator! Before you sleep, as you awaken, and before you nibble, your Whys will encourage you. Armed with the knowledge you are about to absorb, the How is easy.

My mother always said, "In order to succeed, you first need a wishbone, then a backbone."

Your Wishbone – Your Goal

Now is the time to set your own, achievable goals, to really think about what you wish to achieve. This is a contract with yourself!

"Nothing happens unless first a dream."
— Carl Sandburg

When it comes to your body, what are your dreams? That you will fit into those tight slacks? That your thighs will look great in your bathing suit? Or simply that you won't see that ripply fat on your thighs.

Be specific!

Record in your Positive Progress Diary (pages 122–125) what is important to you. Do you prefer to focus on your weight? Are you more interested in your dress size, or just in how you look – your "Reflection Reaction"?

Be realistic!

If your initial wishes and goals are beyond the achievable (too much, too soon), you will be discouraged when you fall short and you may even give up. That just won't do! You cannot change your bone structure or your weight but you can become an improved you!

Set deadlines!

Once you've established realistic goals, set realistic deadlines for yourself – not vague hopes, but real commitments "today", "this week". Make the pledge that you'll look good in your new, short skirt next month. Deadlines "keep you honest" and on track.

Your Backbone – Your Commitment

The trick is commitment! You have already decided to change your lifestyle; all you need to do is commit yourself to a few, new habits. With practice, these will become your routine.

"We first make our habits, and then our habits make us." — John Dryden

Be your own boss!

Many of your habits are part of your life, not because you've consciously adopted them, but because you passively acquired them. Don't let the rest of your life be influenced by subconscious behavioural patterns. As "creatures of habit", our habits should be a part of our lives not by coincidence, but by informed decision! Single out habits that are not in your best interests. If you can identify your patterns of action (or inaction), half the battle is won! Actively plan a new response for each situation. If you can't resist a cake when you pass the bakery, take another route!

Always look to the broader picture!

As you reach for dessert, think instead how much happier you'll be tomorrow weighing less. Make your priority the greater long term pleasure of looking and feeling much better. You control your tastes; they don't control you.

Be patient! Persevere!

Don't expect your body to be transformed after only a few days. Remember, it took you years to acquire the figure you now have; it will be a few weeks before the improvement is really apparent. Set small, incremental goals for each day and week. If you are overweight, you must lose that weight slowly and steadily over several months. A good goal is to lose about 1 kg (2 lb) a week; don't be discouraged by a plateau or even a 0.5 or 1 kg (1 or 2 lb) increase on any given day, such fluctuation is quite natural.

Always visualize the new you!

Pretend you are that svelte silhouette that you wish for now! How would you feel and act? You would consciously and unconsciously feel and act differently, adopting new and healthy habits. You would truly enjoy your body and feel good about yourself. You would eat healthy, nourishing, tasty foods, not junky fats. You would enjoy showing off your cellulite-free self by exercising regularly. You would plan your activities around interests other than eating. At a movie you would concentrate on the film, forgetting the buttered popcorn. At a buffet you would taste, not overeat. "Think Thin Thighs"! If in your mind you reinforce your goal, you will live that goal in all of your actions and you will have new, positive habits to make your goal come true in every sense.

Life is choice

With this book, you now have a plan. Don't let yourself ever become discouraged. Take action and keep it up! It is easier to make comprehensive changes in diet and exercise than to make only moderate ones. Why? Because if you make only moderate changes in lifestyle – giving up one fattening food, such as ice cream – you actually have the worst of both worlds. You feel deprived because you cannot eat what you think you want, but the changes are not enough to change your body significantly or to make you look and feel better. Without full commitment, you will not get positive reinforcement. On the other hand, with commitment, you will make all the necessary changes in your lifestyle, and you will be rewarded by feeling and looking better. Take my word for it: the benefits you quickly reap will far outweigh any transient feelings of deprivation! You are free to choose your lifestyle. You are free to become the person you want to be.

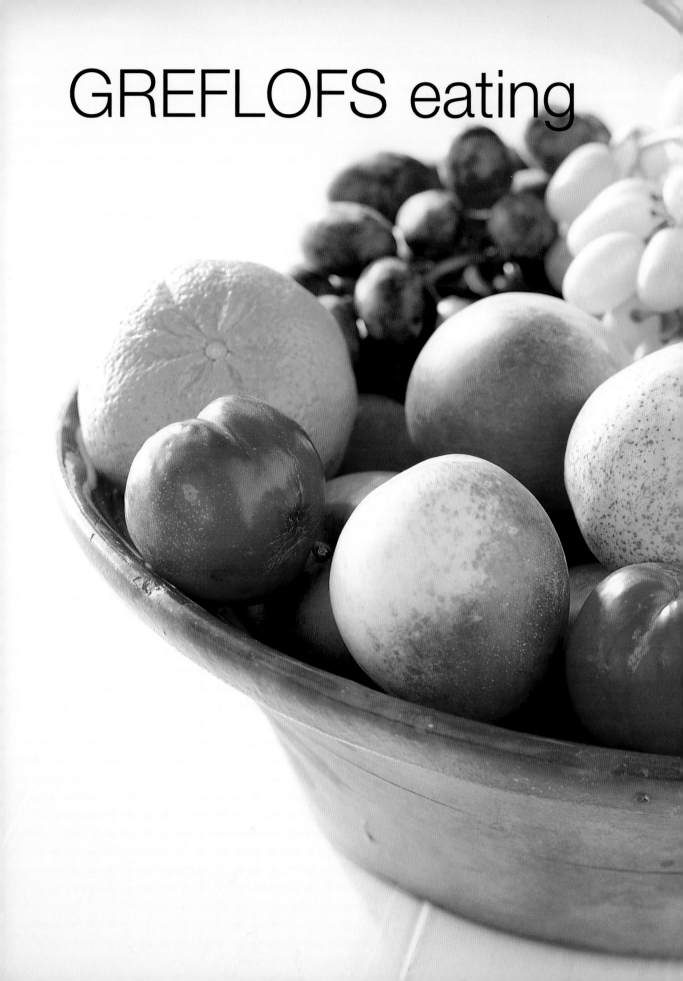

GREFLOFS eating

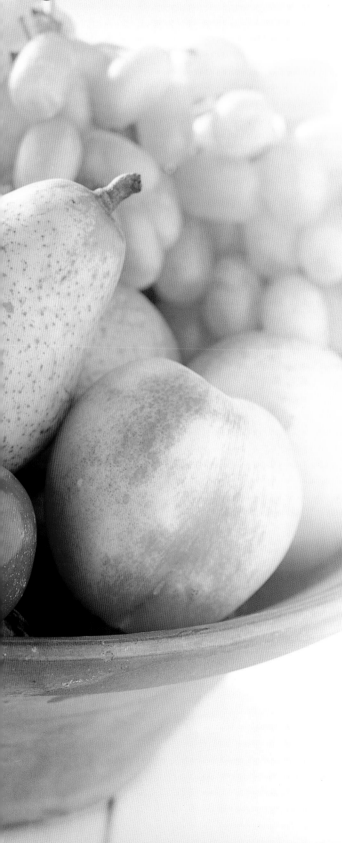

– great food, low fat, sugar free!

You are what you eat. Your body's silhouette is a product of what goes into your mouth. With my programme, you can eat fabulous foods that make you feel and look fantastic, full of energy, and satisfied. The trick is knowledge – understanding which foods you should choose and when you should best eat them. The recipes that follow have been analysed for their nutritional content – energy is measured in kilocalories (kcals); protein, fat and carbohydrate (CHO) are measured in grams (g).

Eating well will become a part of your life. "Diets" always fail because they make you feel deprived, hungry and bored. Telling yourself that you are "on a diet" instantly makes you crave the foods you are supposed to avoid. And a "diet", labelled in your mind as such, is always temporary. You cannot wait to be "off" the diet to eat all the foods you "gave up" – those very foods that made you heavier to begin with! Forget dieting! Instead you can enjoy three meals a day – and several snacks, too. Your hunger will always be satiated.

You need not change your lifestyle. You can still eat out with friends and eat normal meals with your family. You will simply make educated choices about what enters your body. Knowledge is power. You will uncover the "hidden enemies", so you can avoid detrimental foods while enjoying delicious meals.

The GREFLOFS Plan

This is the new GREFLOFS plan that offers you the gift of your ideal weight and increased vigour. You will really enjoy this new way of eating. There are no rigid rules, only concepts based on medical science and common sense. And you need not purchase expensive, special foods. Your neighbourhood grocery store has everything you need.

Your Goal:
To become healthier, energized, and cellulite-free.

1 Limit fats
- Use only unsaturated vegetable oils in limited amounts
- Avoid saturated animal fat
- Avoid fat and salt combinations

2 Avoid extra sugar
- Use artificial sweeteners
- Avoid fat and sugar together

3 The fibre feast: eat more fruits and vegetables

4 Prefer protein

5 Avoid alcohol

6 Graze
- Eat snacks and smaller meals
- Don't eat a large meal late at night
- Eat slowly
- Eat when you are hungry and only when you are hungry

7 Water is wonderful

8 Vitamin vitality: each day take:
Vitamin E (d-alpha-tocopherol)   400 IU
Vitamin C (ascorbic acid) 1000–6000 mg
Calcium   1200–1500 mg

Add years to your life and life to your years

1 Limit Fattening Fats!

We eat more fats today than ever before in history. Why our attraction to fat? We all know that fat gives a richer taste and a creamy texture so that food slithers down easily as we eat. Now we know that there is actually a brain hormone "galanin" which regulates our desire for fat. Dr Sarah Leibowitz at The Rockefeller University showed that when galanin was introduced into animals' brains, they chose to eat more fatty foods and, even worse, that fat was more easily converted directly to body fat. Galanin is released when we eat fat: the more fat we eat, the more galanin we make, and the more fat we crave – a real vicious cycle! Dr Leibowitz showed that animals with a diet consisting of more than 40 per cent fat (approximately a typical British or American diet) had twice as much galanin as those whose diet consisted of less than 20 per cent.

A diet consisting of 15–20 per cent fat is optimal. What does this mean? If you weigh 130 lb (59 kg), you should eat no more than 32 g of fat per day (equal to 288 kilocalories (kcals), since fat has a whopping 9 kcals per gram, in contrast with protein and carbohydrate with only 4 kcals per gram!). Eating this lower quantity of fat not only limits galanin, but also reduces atherosclerosis (thereby decreasing heart attacks and strokes) as well as some forms of cancer.

Fat is fattening

How can we limit fats? With a little knowledge, it's actually easy.

1. Eat only unsaturated fats – that is, fats that are liquid at room temperature, such as vegetable oils (coconut oil and palm oil are the exceptions; both are saturated fats). **Monounsaturated** fats (such as olive oil) are preferable to **polyunsaturated** fats, because they don't raise blood cholesterol levels. However, certain polyunsaturated fats found in fish oils ("**omega-3 fatty acids**", especially high in salmon, mackerel, herring and trout) are healthy because they help prevent excessive blood clotting (thereby decreasing the incidence of heart disease and strokes).

Avoid **saturated** fats that are solid at room temperature, such as the fat on meat and poultry, butter, lard and cheese. Choose margarines made from vegetable oils, preferably the softer ones in the tub, since they contain less saturated fat.

2. Cook in non-stick pans without fats. Substitute fat-free or low-fat ingredients for butter and oil. See Cooking Tips on page 27.

3. Especially avoid foods with salt and fat. Salt makes high-fat foods taste better, so we eat more! Can you ever eat only one potato chip or only one peanut? All adults should avoid extra salt! Salt causes water to accumulate between fat cells. Your cellulite not only looks worse, but it becomes worse since blood flow is slowed. With time, the capillary structure can actually change to slow your blood flow and your metabolism. Even if you don't salt your food, be aware of hidden salts in the foods you eat. Cheese is a particular villain, as are canned soups, canned vegetables, soft drinks, diet sodas, and luncheon meats. Be careful to ask for no salt when you are ordering in restaurants!

Re-educate your palate. Discover exciting herbs and spices like pepper, dill, oregano, tarragon, garlic, onion, cumin, curry, parsley, sage, rosemary and thyme.

4. Learn where there are hidden fats, so that you can avoid them. Realize which foods are the culprits. We all know that red meat has fat, but did you know that animals are extra-fattened purposefully before slaughter, and that extra fat is added to hamburgers and hot dogs? The danger is the readily available "fast food" such as French fries in which 13 g (½ oz) of fat (250 kcals) is added to a potato containing no fat and only 60 kcals! There is

"hidden fat" in many supposedly healthy foods like granola breakfast bars, yogurt, imitation ice cream, non-dairy coffee whitener, and baked goods like cookies and cakes. Read the labels before you buy and choose lower-fat foods. You can purchase low-fat foods that taste just as good!

2 Avoid Extra Sugar

Our bodies do not physiologically "need" sugar. Humans have only consumed sugar for a brief span in history. Refined sugar did not exist anywhere in the world until 700 AD. (The Bible does not even mention sugar!) Refined sugar should be labelled "Hazardous to Your Health". The reason is that sugar directly causes the pancreas to release **insulin**; and insulin inhibits the breakdown of fat and facilitates the storage of fat. Therefore sugar makes fat even more fattening! Furthermore, excess sugar is converted to and stored as fat!

Biologically, no one is a "sugar addict"; any "addiction" is psychological. Sugar tastes good. What is even worse, foods that contain both sugar and fat are the best-tasting foods! This is precisely the dreadful combination in the foods we crave: chocolate, ice cream, cheesecake, cookies, cakes. About 48 per cent of the calories in these foods are from FAT! Fatty hot dogs are bad enough, but adding ketchup (which contains sugar) is even worse. The sugar stimulates insulin, which signals the body to store the fat and excess sugar in the fat deposits. For women, this means more cellulite. You will learn later in this chapter how to avoid these downfalls.

Sugar makes fat more fattening

Give children nutritious diets with few or no refined sugars and minimal fats. Especially in young children, inordinate weight gain can promote the formation of more fat cells. Once they have been created, these fat cells are on the body forever, ready to absorb all extra fat eaten and making weight gain later in life physiologically easier.

3 Enjoy The Fibre Feast: Fruits and Vegetables

Believe it or not, you can actually lose fat and cellulite by eating huge amounts of certain foods. The trick is to eat natural "hard" foods that have bulk. You will enjoy tasting, chewing and swallowing, and you will feel so full that you could not possibly eat one more bite of anything for hours! These magical, healthy foods are high-fibre fruits and vegetables.

Eat more to weigh less!

Fibre is the part of food that cannot be digested – but that does fill your stomach. Soluble fibres attract and hold water in the digestive tract; they actually gain volume in your stomach and intestine! Insoluble fibres add bulk; they are not even absorbed! Both types of fibre delay digestion and emptying, to make you feel satiated for a longer time. The more fibre you eat early in a meal or early in the day, the less hungry you are later on. And fibre actually decreases your body's absorption of carbohydrates (including sugar), and fat. Less insulin is released so less fat is stored.

Fibre is filling

Fibre is complex carbohydrate, which gives 4 kcals of energy per gram absorbed. The best fibres are those that are the most bulky, and therefore most filling, with the fewest kilocalories, and with the lowest insulin-releasing response. You will feel satiated if you eat a serving of 250 g (8 oz) of cabbage, cucumber or spinach (each only about 15 kcals), or strawberries or melon (each only about 45 kcals). But avoid those fibres which induce insulin release.

If you are a vegetarian who eats no animal protein, be sure to eat both wholegrain cereals and legumes, such as peas, beans and lentils, so that you get all of the essential amino acids. (Cereals are low in the essential amino acid lysine, and legumes are similiarly low in methionine, so your diet must include both.)

The Fibre Feast: Vegetables

You may eat an unlimited amount of the following raw or steamed vegetables with tasty herbal seasoning, but do not add salt, butter or sauce:

artichokes	green beans
asparagus	greens
aubergine	lentils*
bamboo shoots	lettuce
beans*	mangetout
bean sprouts	okra
broccoli	onion
Brussels sprouts	parsley
butternut squash	peppers
cabbage	(red, green or yellow)
cauliflower	radish
celery	spinach
chicory	sweet potatoes*
courgette	tomatoes
cucumber	turnips
fennel	watercress

*These vegetables can only be enjoyed cooked. The serving size should be limited to 50 g (2 oz), as they are relatively high in kilocalories.

Insulin-releasing fibres to avoid

bananas
beetroot
carrots
corn and corn flakes
processed grains (white rice, white bread)
raisins
white potatoes

The Fibre Feast: Fruits

You may eat one serving of the following delicious fruits, equal to:

1 apple
2 plums
1 peach or nectarine
125 g/4 oz fresh pineapple

½ grapefruit or 125 ml/4 floz unsweetened grapefruit juice
125 g (4 oz) blueberries, strawberries, or raspberries
125 g (4 oz) cherries
125 g (4 oz) kiwis

½ cantaloupe
¼ honeydew melon
6 mm/ ¼ inch slice watermelon

A word about cooking: The more you refine, grind, or soften vegetables or fruit, the less filling they become. The reason is simple: the carbohydrate content of these fibre-rich foods is broken down into sugar during the process of digestion. The more refined the carbohydrate, the quicker the sugars enter your body, and the more insulin is released. Also, overcooking soluble fibre (especially oats, beans and brown rice) decreases their fibre content.

Steam vegetables very lightly, so that they are slightly crunchy when you eat them, and serve fruits raw in order to preserve both their taste and their texture – and to give yourself their full advantage!

4 Prefer Protein

While sugar and refined carbohydrate cause insulin release, protein stimulates the release of "glucagon", a hormone whose action balances insulin. While insulin increases the storage of fat and inhibits the breakdown of fat, glucagon promotes the breakdown of previously stored fat. And glucagon levels stay elevated for a while after a high protein meal so that stored fat continues to be mobilized.

The other great advantage of protein is that it is very satisfying. Protein sends a direct signal to your brain to decrease your appetite. You cannot eat more than one or two portions of chicken or fish at one meal – but you can easily consume piles of fatty foods like French fries. It is better to eat protein at the beginning of a meal and early in the day. Restaurants know that you eat less if you eat protein first, so they stimulate your appetite by first serving white bread and alcohol.

"Square meals often make round people."
— E. Joseph Cossman

Several books have been written about so-called food combining. Their basic philosophy is that the human body cannot digest protein and starch at the same time. Though it is true that starch digestion begins in the mouth with the action of saliva and protein digestion begins in the stomach, mixing these foods does not change digestion in any way. There is no scientific evidence that the way foods are mixed alters their assimilation.

However, if you limit the variety of tastes at one meal, you automatically eat less. I call this the "Christmas Dinner Syndrome". You eat the main course of turkey with stuffing, potatoes and vegetables until you are stuffed and can't eat a bite more. Then the dessert appears and, of course, you cannot resist. However, if dessert were still more turkey with stuffing, potatoes and vegetables, you most certainly would not have that "other bite"! I recommend that for breakfast you choose between a protein (an egg white omelette) or a carbohydrate (such as wholegrain rice, bran muffins or Slimming French Toast, page 33), with or without a Fibre Feast vegetable or salad, and that for lunch and dinner you eat a serving of protein with Fibre Feast vegetables.

5 Avoid Alcohol

When you are actively trying to lose weight and cellulite, avoid or minimize alcohol. Alcohol provides no nutrition – in fact, it requires extra work by the liver to be metabolized, and it has 7 kcals per gram – almost as much as the 9 kcals per gram contributed by fat! Alcohol also causes some insulin release (but less than a serving of corn or a slice of white bread).

Even more unfortunate, alcohol does not satisfy your appetite at all. Actually, it makes you more likely to indulge in high-fat snacks, like those served in bars and at parties. Wine at dinner enhances the taste of food and impairs our judgment, so that we eat more.

If you really want to indulge, red wine is the most acceptable (with 137 kcals per 175g/ 6 oz glass). One glass daily of some red wines may, in fact, decrease atherosclerosis. Avoid beer (150 kcals per glass) and dessert wine (240 kcals per glass), since they both cause a rapid increase in insulin. It is advisable to drink alcohol only with or after eating, because when the stomach is full, the absorption of alcohol is slowed.

6 Graze

Humans evolved as "grazing" beings. Look at infants: they eat small amounts every four hours, not huge amounts two or three times each day. We did not start to eat three meals a day until the Industrial Revolution, when life had to revolve around the factory schedule. Now we are made to feel guilty eating snacks. Actually, eating many small meals is the healthiest way to eat – as long as the snacks are not processed, fatty, fast foods but healthy Happy Hunger Helpers!

Grazing is an especially good way to eat for nervous eaters (who can munch all the time), and for compulsive eaters (who no longer have to "gorge"). The best schedule to adopt is "breakfast like a king, lunch like a queen, and dine like a pauper", with a high-fibre snack

between each meal (in mid-morning and mid-to late afternoon, but at least one hour before dinner). It is especially good not to eat a large meal within three hours of going to bed, since you will not really burn any of those kilocalories while you sleep! It is acceptable, however, to have a healthy, high-fibre snack one hour before sleeping.

Unfortunately, our modern lifestyle and schedules usually do not quite permit such a "royal diet", but you can try to eat more filling protein early in the day, since that helps curb your appetite later on. The advantage of eating snacks between main meals is that you do not begin a meal famished. When you start a meal starving, you tend to eat a lot of food rapidly. You cannot begin to feel satiated until at least 20 minutes after the first bite, but by that time you might have already eaten far more than you need!

Try to eat slowly

Give your stomach time to fill, and your brain time to turn off your hunger, when you eat a whole meal!

Eat only when you are hungry

If you are not hungry at a meal or snack-time, eat very little or drink a glass of water. But if you do choose to skip a meal or snack, be sure not to let yourself become "famished". Always carry a small bag of Happy Hunger Helpers – healthy, high-fibre snacks – to nibble (see opposite page).

There is another physiological advantage to snacking. Remember the brain hormone galanin, which increases our craving for fat? Galanin is released when your brain detects fat in the blood, either after eating fat or when your body breaks down fat in "starvation" – that is, whenever you have not eaten for more than six to eight hours. If you graze, eating smaller amounts more often, you decrease the production of galanin, which actually decreases any craving that you might have for fat.

7 Water is Wonderful

Water is the best beverage! It has no kcals, no fat, and no chemical additives, and can be marvellous help for curbing hunger. Thirty minutes before each meal, drink a room temperature glass of sparkling* or still water (with a squeezed lemon, lime or orange sliver for taste and elegance). Or have an Italian "canarino" – a cup of hot water flavoured with a slice of lemon. (This is great when you are hungry between meals.) If you are famished, eat a fibre-rich food with a glass of water before your meal. The fibre expands, so you will feel satiated before you begin your meal.

Here's a special secret: drinking water during a meal can be a disaster. It allows you to swallow before you have fully chewed. You eat more with less enjoyment! Especially avoid ice-cold water, since it actually turns on your digestive enzymes and increases your hunger. Drink no more than one glass of water with your meal, but drink as much as you want between meals.

* If you drink bottled fizzy water, read the label. Some contain calcium, which is good. Avoid those that contain unwanted sodium.

8 Vitamin Vitality

The astonishing fact about vitamins is not only that small amounts prevent deficiency diseases, but also that extra supplements markedly improve health. Vitamins C and E may directly help to reduce cellulite. Also, as you limit dairy products to decrease saturated fats, a calcium supplement is advisable.

It is not possible to get a sufficient amount of vitamins E and C from your diet alone. You would have to take 44 tablespoons of sunflower oil, equal to 5,275 kcals of pure fat, and consume more than 100 oranges, or many pounds of peppers or blackcurrants! Vitamins C and E are free-radical quenching antioxidants that protect us against ultraviolet radiation, chemical pollutants, ionizing radiation,

Happy Hunger Helpers

Happy Hunger Helpers are great snacks you can enjoy between meals! Here are a few:

1 Carbonated water mixed with grapefruit, orange, pineapple, apple or cranberry juice.

2 Hot or cold water with a slice of lemon, lime, or orange, or with a tablespoon of cider or balsamic vinegar (and artificial sweetener if you wish).

3 Sticks of courgette, celery and turnip. Store these standing in a glass in the refrigerator with a little water in the bottom, or carry them to work in a zip-lock plastic bag (after washing the vegetables without drying).

4 Cut slices of red, yellow or green pepper, cucumber, cherry tomatoes, lettuce leaves, and/or radishes.

5 Washed and trimmed string beans, runner beans, asparagus.

6 Cut thin slices of orange, pear, apple, peach and chunks of pineapple or melon.

7 Air-popped popcorn made with seasonings, with no butter or salt. (If you must add butter, use low-calorie, low-fat margarine.) Try seasonings such as cumin, cinnamon with artificial sweetener, curry, onion, garlic, dill, coriander, sage, thyme. (Although corn does cause insulin release, a large bowl of popcorn which gives four generous servings is equivalent to only about an eighth of a serving of corn.)

8 Sugar-free sweets.

9 Wheat cakes.

10 Non-sweetened cereals: especially puffed wheat, bran flakes, or shredded wheat.

thermal burns and many kinds of cancer. They also strengthen the immune system, and help prevent atherosclerosis, thereby decreasing heart attacks and strokes. If these reasons are not enough, the fact that vitamins C and E help fight cellulite most certainly warrants taking them. Both vitamins C and E are important in the remodelling of collagen and can help to inhibit the thickening of the connective tissue sacs that package the fat cells in our cellulite. Less thickening means less cellulite.

Both of these vitamins also protect against possible skin tissue damage. Aerobic exercise generates free radicals which, in turn, damage muscle tissue. The benefits of aerobic exercise, essential for a cellulite-free body, are thereby limited. By quenching free radicals, vitamins C and E actually increase exercise tolerance. And they protect your skin from sun damage-though you should always use a high SPF sunscreen (greater than SPF 20) when you exercise outside.

Every adult should take 1000–6000 mg of vitamin C daily, as capsules, effervescent tablets placed in water, or ascorbic acid crystals (1 teaspoon equals 3000 mg) mixed into water or juice. (If this upsets your stomach, take vitamins after food or use a slow-release kind.)

Most vitamin E on the market is synthetic, a mixture of 32 isomers, only one of which (d-alpha-tocopherol) has significantly higher biological potency. Avoid vitamin E labelled mixed tocopherols or dl-alpha tocopherol. The best form of vitamin E is natural vitamin E – d-alpha tocopherol or d-alpha tocopheryl acetate (an oil) or d-alpha tocopheryl succinate (a dry powder). Every adult should take 400 IU per day (in capsule form) to help live a longer, healthier and cellulite-free life.

Calcium

Most of us are aware that calcium is important to our bones, particularly to prevent osteoporosis in our later years. The Recommended Daily Allowance (RDA) for women is 1200 mg of calcium per day,

increasing to 1500 mg per day after the age of 50 years. Pregnant women should take 1200–1600 mg per day (check with your doctor).

How can we get enough calcium if we limit our intake of dairy products to avoid their high fat content? Since foods with calcium are relatively high in kcals, I recommend instead taking calcium supplements. Calcium citrate, which is better absorbed than calcium carbonate, is best. Supplements such as dolomite and bone meal should be avoided since they may contain lead or other possibly toxic elements. With all these choices, a cellulite-fighter can easily consume sufficient calcium – it just takes planning.

GREFLOFS Recipe Replacements

Use	Instead of
ground pepper chopped garlic dill coriander grated ginger	salt
poultry	meat, in meatloaf and chilli
low-fat yogurt	mayonnaise sour cream
skimmed milk (fat-free or 1% fat) evaporated skimmed milk	cream
arrowroot	flour (as thickener)
butternut squash	spaghetti
puréed fruit (eg. apple sauce)	butter in cake recipes* oil in muffins
puréed prunes	butter in brownies oil in brownies
egg whites	eggs**
grated celery courgette	breadcrumbs
chicken stock	butter or oil to sauté

* Use the same amount of fruit as the amount of fat required in the recipe.
** If several eggs are required, add only 1 yolk.

GREFLOFS Cooking Tips

1 Always choose cookware with non-stick surfaces. Treat yourself to the special new pans available, such as a frying pan with concentric grooves for grilling. Sometimes the instructions advise "conditioning" the non-stick surface with a little vegetable cooking oil, then wiping off with a paper towel. You can also use a short squirt of non-fat, no-calorie cooking spray for frying or sautéing.

2 To replace the flavour that fat gives, season foods with a teaspoon of an acidic seasoning such as white wine, a squeeze of fresh lemon, lime or orange juice, or a few drops of balsamic vinegar.

3 Create your own sensational low-calorie, low-fat dishes from your favourite high-fat recipes by seasoning without salt and by replacing high-fat or insulin-releasing ingredients with fat-free, non-insulin-releasing ingredients.

4 Always remove the skin from poultry and fish before cooking. (Chicken can be cooked with the skin to keep it juicy, but discard the skin before you add the final seasonings.)

5 Always remove all visible fat from meats, poultry and fish before cooking.

6 Cook mushrooms, tomatoes, green peppers and other vegetables in the microwave for 2 minutes, covered, with a few drops of water in the pan.

7 Instead of sautéing garlic, onion and other vegetables in oil, place in a pan with a small amount of stock, wine or water. Cover tightly and cook gently, until the vegetables are soft (usually only a few minutes).

8 Always thoroughly brown and drain ground, or minced, meat. Then put in a separate bowl and rinse in hot water to remove extra fat.

9 Always purchase the low-fat or fat-free versions of yogurt, cheese, cottage cheese, ricotta, sour cream, skimmed milk and evaporated skimmed milk.

10 Never add breadcrumbs to ground or minced beef or poultry. Breadcrumbs soak in the fat rather than allowing it to drip off.

11 Make croûtons for soups and salads from wholegrain light bread, in the microwave or toaster without adding any butter or margarine.

12 Some recipes require stock. To eliminate fat, make your own! To make vegetable and fish stocks, just simmer a selection of vegetables and herbs or fish heads and bones with herbs in water for 20–30 minutes. Meat and poultry stocks are made by simmering bones (without fat!) for 1–2 hours. Refrigerate overnight and skim off the fat that rises to the surface. You can freeze stock in ice cube trays and use as many cubes as you need.

13 Freshly grated rind and juice from lemons, limes and oranges enhance sauces, toppings and salad dressings.

14 If you lead a hectic lifestyle, you can prepare more than you need of each special low-calorie recipe and freeze the extra. Then you always have a healthy meal ready – easy to heat or microwave.

Vitamin Supplements:

1 Vitamin E: 400 IU/day
d-alpha tocopherol
or
d-alpha tocopheryl
     succinate
or
d-alpha tocopheryl acetate

2 Vitamin C: 1000-6000 mg/day

3 Calcium: 1200 to 1500 mg/day

GREFLOFS Lifestyle Hints

1 Never sit down to a meal famished. Even if you are not hungry, 30 minutes before you plan to eat, drink a large glass of water. Your excessive hunger will be satiated!

2 Eat breakfast, lunch and dinner and two or three snacks.

3 Never, never, never eat between snacks! (With so many snacks, how could you?) This is a joke.

4 Eat only when you are hungry! If you're not hungry enough for a snack, skip it, but be sure not to be famished before your next meal. If you're not hungry at mealtimes, eat only a little.

5 Slow down! Always eat sitting down, actively savouring every bite as you chew. Try to eat more slowly than everyone else.

6 Designate a specific place to eat, at home or at work. This will help you break the habit of eating on the run.

7 Avoid eating in front of television, at the movies, or as a sports spectator. This diminishes any habitual, involuntary eating.

8 Cut your food into small pieces; take small bites; chew each bite at least 10 times.

9 Taste your food! Don't add extra salt, especially without tasting first.

10 Fill your salt shakers with other seasonings.

11 Try salads without dressing – or with lemon or balsamic vinegar and herbs only.

12 Fry in non-stick pans with low-calorie, non-fat cooking spray instead of butter or oil.

13 Any time you are hungry between meals, delay. Brush your teeth* or chew sugar-free gum. Wait 20 minutes and do some Pressometrics, tidy your desk or read an article. You will probably not even be hungry any longer – a scientifically proven fact!

14 If you are still hungry after a 20-minute delay, drink a large glass of hot or cold water (flavoured with lemon, lime or orange juice), then wait another 20 minutes.

15 If you are still hungry, snack on a healthy Happy Hunger Helper.

16 If you really have a particular food craving, first follow hints 13 to 15. If you still absolutely must eat that food, allow yourself a few small bites. Throw the rest away, even before you eat. Do not let just a few minutes of breaking your eating plan become an excuse to binge.

17 If you live alone, throw out all the fatty junk food you have immediately! If your family or room mate absolutely must eat fattening foods, then keep them all in a separate place.

18 Never go food shopping when you're feeling hungry.

19 Shop smart. Do not even buy the foods that you now know to avoid. It is easier to have willpower for a short time in the supermarket than all the time at home.

20 Socialize with friends at places where you do not eat. Walk in the park or in your neighbourhood, window shop, or visit a museum instead of planning meetings over breakfast, lunch, tea, cocktails, dinner, or dessert.

21 When eating in restaurants, always specify that any sauces, sour cream, butter, margarine, and salad dressings be served "on the side", so that you, yourself, control any extra fat you might eat.

22 If you are served a large portion in a restaurant, simply decide immediately to eat only half. Divide the food into this half-portion mentally as soon as the plate is placed in front of you. (You can always take the other half home, if you wish.)

23 Avoid buffets! If you really have to go, use a salad or a dessert plate instead of a large dinner plate – or, better still, use a saucer! (The so-called Saucer Diet is to eat no more than will fit conveniently on a saucer at each meal!)

24 Never go out hungry, especially for lunch, cocktails or dinner!

25 Remember that the food from other people's plates has kilocalories too, and so do leftovers!

26 Eat only foods you like! Do not eat just to be polite. It is better to throw away those unnecessary kilocalories than to have them stored on your hips!

27 Always keep healthy Happy Hunger Helpers nearby, ready for snack attacks.

28 If you are a nervous nibbler, chew sugar-free gum instead of munching food.

29 Make it a firm policy never to take second helpings!

30 Brush your teeth! Your mother taught you to brush your teeth before bed; I am now suggesting that you also brush your teeth after every meal and after every snack. When your mouth feels really clean, you don't feel like eating more! Always carry your toothbrush with you, and experiment with all the great flavours of many of the toothpastes that you can buy nowadays!

* A note on brushing: use a soft brush; dampen the brush with warm water (which softens it even more) and brush up and down (not across) your teeth. Be sure to brush your gums and even your tongue (especially if you have a problem with bad breath!)

Absolutely forbidden:

- butter and buttery sauces
- all foods fried in oil
- saturated fats on meat and poultry
- other saturated fats (rich cheese, lard)
- all dairy products (except fat-free milk, low-fat yogurt, low-fat ricotta, low-fat cream or cottage cheese)
- extra salt
- extra sugar (including honey)
- nuts and fatty snacks
- bread* (except wholegrain breads)
- white rice**
- refined pasta***

* Wholegrain breads can be eaten in limited amounts.
** Brown rice and wholegrain rice can be eaten in limited amounts.
*** Wholegrain pasta can be eaten in limited amounts.

If you absolutely crave sugar:

- use an artificial sweetener
- eat one serving of fruit
- drink a diet soda
- suck a sugar-free sweet
- chew gum
- air pop popcorn and sweeten with artificial sugar and cinnamon
- add to cooked rice: fruit and fruit juice or artificial sugar and cinnamon
- drink a glass of water with 1 tablespoon lemon juice or 1 tablespoon cider vinegar and artificial sweetener. (This drink is really refreshing hot or cold; with vinegar it tastes like apple cider.)
- brush your teeth with a great flavoured toothpaste

Happy Breakfasts

Breakfast is a special treat, something well worth waking up to enjoy!
Breakfast can be the most exciting and variable meal of the day. It can
be so satisfying that you really will not begin to be hungry until lunch
time. Like me, you might prefer a "double" breakfast: 120 ml (4 fl oz)
unsweetened grapefruit or orange juice or 1 serving of a preferred fruit
just after you awaken and the more hearty portion a bit later. Do
something luxuriously different for yourself. For example, treat yourself to
a special tray, so that you can take your breakfast to a cosy, tranquil
place. Giving yourself just a few minutes of enjoyment gives a
psychological jump-start to the day which usually becomes rapidly
hectic in our modern technological age – whether you are in a work
place or at home with your children or other responsibilities.

Make every meal an occasion, a luxurious experience, both aesthetically
and sensually. A real "event" at breakfast can be enjoying your coffee or
tea. Experiment with different blends: treat yourself and your family to a
special coffee-maker or a beautiful teapot. They need not be expensive!
This gift to yourself will symbolize your enjoyment of your new, healthy
eating regime that will lead to a svelte figure with thin thighs. You may
have as much coffee or tea as you want, using low-fat milk and artificial
sweetener if you wish.

The main course of the GREFLOFS breakfast should be one of the following:

1 Wholegrain Rice Banquet (page 31) alone or topped with:
1 portion of preferred fruit
or 1–2 servings of Fibre Feast vegetables (page 22)
or a Super Salad (page 40)

2 Fresh Berry Muffin (page 31) alone or with: a Super Salad
or 1 Light Raisin Bran Muffin (page 32) *or* 1–2 servings of Fibre Feast vegetables
or 1 slice toasted Tsoureki (page 33)
or 1–2 slices of low-calorie wholegrain bread, toasted

3 Gourmet Light Omelette (page 34) of your choice

4 Slimming French Toast (page 33)

5 About 120 g (4 oz) unsweetened cereal, preferably puffed or shredded wheat,
rice or bran flakes with 120 ml (4 fl oz) skimmed milk.

6 A Super Salad of your choice

7 1–3 servings of your favourite Fibre Feast vegetables

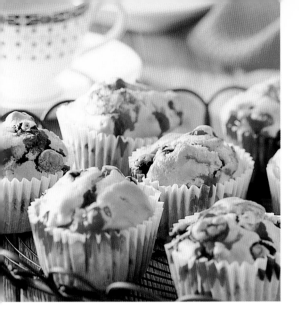

Fresh Berry Muffins

per muffin: 92 kcals • 3 g protein • 2 g fat • 18 g CHO

Makes 12

225 g (8 oz) flour

2 tsp baking powder

⅛ tsp salt

1 egg and 2 egg whites

1¾ tsp artificial sweetener

1 tbs maple syrup

1 tbs vegetable oil

120 ml(4 fl oz) low-fat milk

225 g (8 oz) cranberries or blueberries

1 Sift the flour, baking powder and salt into a bowl.

2 In a separate bowl, beat the egg or egg whites. Add the artificial sweetener, maple syrup, and vegetable oil and mix.

3 To the sifted flour, alternately add the milk and the egg mixture, mixing each addition until smooth.

4 Wash the berries and drain. Mash 50 g (2 oz) and mix into the batter.

5 Stir 1 tablespoon flour into the other berries so that the flour covers each berry. (This prevents the whole berries from falling to the bottom of the batter.) Fold the berries gently into the batter.

6 Spoon the batter into a non-stick deep bun tin or paper cups, filling each section about two-thirds full.

7 Bake in a preheated oven at 190°C (375°F), Gas Mark 5, for 30 minutes.

(Note: These are especially delicious when served warm. Serve alone or with a low-calorie jam; do not add butter or margarine.)

Wholegrain Rice Banquet

per portion: 145 kcals • 3 g protein • 0 g fat • 35 g CHO

Serves 8

300 g (10 oz) brown basmati rice

50 g (2 oz) wild rice

850 ml (1½ pints) vegetable stock (water saved after steaming vegetables)

1 Cook the rice slowly in boiling vegetable stock for 40–45 minutes until tender.

2 Store the rice in the refrigerator for a quick, hearty breakfast.

3 Remove 50–75 g (2–3 oz) and heat in a microwave for 40 seconds.

4 Enjoy alone or top with 1 portion of your favourite Fibre Feast fruit (page 23)
  or 1–2 servings of Fibre Feast vegetables (page 22)
  or a Super Salad (page 40)
  or low-calorie cinnamon sugar (page 33)
  or low-calorie jam of your choice

Light Raisin Bran Muffins

per muffin: 130 kcals • 4 g protein • 3 g fat • 20 g CHO

Makes 6

1 tbs vegetable oil

1 tbs soft dark brown sugar

1 tbs maple syrup

1¼ tsp artificial sweetener

1 egg and 1 egg white, beaten

120 ml (4 fl oz) skimmed milk

120 g (4 oz) self-raising flour

1 tsp baking powder

½ tsp bicarbonate of soda

½ tsp salt

2 tbs bran

75 g (3 oz) raisins

1 Combine the oil, sugar, syrup, artificial sweetener, beaten eggs and milk in a large bowl. Mix thoroughly.

2 Sift in the flour, baking powder, bicarbonate of soda and salt. Stir very lightly until the ingredients are just mixed.

3 Sprinkle in the bran and raisins and mix well.

4 Spoon the batter into a non-stick deep bun tin or paper cups, filling each section about two-thirds full.

5 Bake in a preheated oven at 190°C (375°F), Gas Mark 6, for 15 minutes, until well risen and firm to the touch.

(Note: These are especially delicious when served warm. Serve alone or with a low-calorie jam; do not add butter or margarine.)

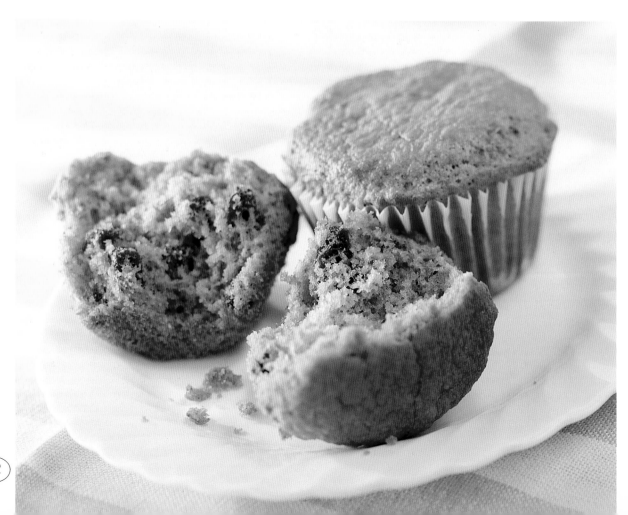

Tsoureki (Greek Easter Bread)

per slice: 124 kcals • 4 g protein • 2 g fat • 31 g CHO

**Makes 2 loaves,
14 slices each**

*40 g (1½ oz) diet
unsalted margarine*

*225 ml (8 fl oz)
skimmed milk*

175 ml (6 fl oz) water

800 g (1¾ lb) flour

5 tbs sugar

2 tbs active dry yeast

1 tsp salt

2 eggs

1 egg white

1 In a saucepan, heat the margarine, milk and water.

2 In a mixer, combine 700 g (1½ lb) of flour with the sugar, yeast and salt. Slowly add in the margarine mixture.

3 Add the eggs and egg white to the mixture. Run on a low speed for about 10 minutes, until everything is completely mixed.

4 Slowly add in the remaining flour, a little at a time, to ensure the dough does not stick.

5 Place the dough in a large non-stick bowl or one coated with vegetable oil cooking spray, cover it with a cloth, and put it in a warm place to rise. Let it rise until it has doubled in size, (about 45 minutes to 1 hour).

6 Remove the dough from the bowl and place it on a floured board. Cut it in half, knead it, and then roll each half into a 23 cm (9 inch) log. Put each half in a loaf tin.

7 Cover the dough and let it rise for another 30–45 minutes. It should be over the top of the loaf tin.

8 Bake the bread in a preheated oven, 180°C (350°F), Gas Mark 4, for 30 minutes.

Cinnamon Swirl

per slice: 147 kcals • 4 g protein • 2 g fat • 31 g CHO

Makes 2 loaves, 14 slices each

Follow the recipe above, but just before allowing dough to rise a second time, stretch out the dough until flat and brush on a small amount of margarine with a pastry brush. Combine 5½ tsp artificial sweetener and 3 tsp cinnamon and sprinkle over the top. Start at one end of the dough and roll it into a cylinder. Place the dough, seam side down, in a loaf tin. Let it rise for another 45 minutes as described above, and bake in a preheated oven, 180°C (350°F), Gas Mark 4 for 30 minutes.

Slimming French Toast

per slice: 62 kcals • 7 g protein • 0 g fat • 8 g CHO

Serves 1

2 egg whites

1 tsp skimmed milk

¼ tsp vanilla essence

1 slice low-calorie, wholegrain bread

1 Beat the egg whites with a fork in a flat soup dish.

2 Add the milk and vanilla. Beat again.

3 Soak one slice of bread in the egg mixture for at least 2 minutes on each side, until the whole egg mixture is absorbed.

4 Cook in a non-stick frying pan, turning after the edges of the first side are brown.

(Note: Serve with low-calorie maple syrup, low-calorie jams, or with Low-Calorie Cinnamon Sugar, below.)

Low-Calorie Cinnamon Sugar

Combine ¼ teaspoon artificial sweetener with ¼ teaspoon cinnamon. Mix well and sprinkle on Slimming French Toast.

Gourmet Light Omelette

per portion: 32 kcals • 6 g protein • 0 g fat • 1 g CHO

Serves 3

6 egg whites

1 tbs skimmed milk or water

1 tbs chopped parsley

pepper

chopped or grated vegetables, to fill

fresh parsley, to garnish

1 Beat the egg whites with the milk or water. (Egg whites are best beaten when at room temperature.)

2 Season the beaten eggs with parsley and pepper.

3 Pour into a hot, non-stick frying pan. Cook on a low heat, turning the pan so that the soft top is cooked. Continue until the edges are almost dry.

4 Meanwhile, in a non-stick pan, lightly cook any combination of chopped or grated vegetables you like; especially delicious are tomato, red or green peppers, spinach, mushrooms, onions and courgettes (see below).

5 Put the vegetables in a line along the centre of the omelette and fold in the two edges. Turn over and cook until light brown. Garnish with parsley.

Alternative omelette fillings

1 Prepare one omelette as above.

2 Select one of the fillings below and prepare according to instructions.

3 Place the filling in a line along the centre of the omelette and fold in the edges. Turn over and cook until light brown. Garnish with parsley.

El Paso Omelette

per portion: 29 kcals • 6 g protein • 0 g fat • 1 g CHO

Serves 3

1 x 20 cm (8 inch) courgette, grated

2 tbs chicken stock

1 garlic clove, crushed

1 spring onion, finely chopped

pinch of oregano

pinch of pepper

fresh parsley, to garnish

1 Cook courgette in a pan with chicken stock, garlic and onion.

2 Put in omelette and garnish.

Tomato-Basil Omelette

per portion: 40 kcals • 7 g protein • 0 g fat • 3 g CHO

Serves 3

3 large tomatoes, peeled

1 spring onion, chopped

1 tsp dried basil

1 tsp finely chopped fresh basil

½ garlic clove, finely chopped

pinch of pepper

fresh parsley, to garnish

1 Cut tomatoes into thin wedges, collecting juice in a non-stick pan.

2 Add seasonings. Stir over low heat until soft. Put in omelette.

Light Apple-Blueberry Pancakes

per pancake: 100 kcals • 3 g protein • 0 g fat • 23 g CHO

Serves 10 *(large pancakes)*

225 g (8 oz) wholewheat flour

½ tsp baking soda

500 ml (17 fl oz) skimmed milk

225 g (8 oz) apple sauce, unsweetened

½ tsp cinnamon

120 g (4 oz) blueberries

1 Mix flour and baking soda. Add milk slowly, stirring to a smooth consistency.

2 Mix in apple sauce and cinnamon.

3 Add blueberries. Stir to distribute evenly.

4 Cook in non-stick pan without oil until the edges are dry. Turn and cook until golden.

Great Light Lunches

Lunch can be the most creative meal of the day. There are so many options! A salad is refreshing and filling; adding soup makes a more substantial meal. Also, each of the starters described on pages 47–50 makes an elegant lunch. You can "mix and match" soups, salads, sandwiches, starters, or special vegetable dishes. With the GREFLOFS plan, you may have as much green leafy salad or crudités as you wish with one portion of chicken or fish or with 120 g (4 oz) rice or 50 g (2 oz) pasta, or with a sweet potato or baked potato. With these light lunches, you really can control your weight and your silhouette!

The very best way of eating is to eat your "dinner" at midday and your "lunch" in the evening. Unfortunately, our schedules and our social and business obligations do not always permit this. If, indeed, you do eat a large meal during the day, be sure to take smaller portions and choose lighter fare in the evenings.

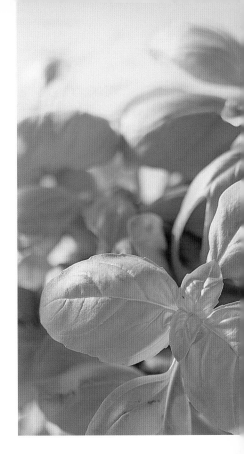

Special Sandwiches

per sandwich using 1 small pitta bread: 228 kcals • 11 g protein • 1 g fat • 47 g CHO

pitta bread

chopped hard-boiled egg whites

celery

cucumber

dill pickles

green, red or yellow pepper

palm hearts

lettuce

red or green cabbage

tomato

turnip greens

watercress

coriander

courgettes

other Fibre Feast vegetables

fresh parsley and coriander, to garnish

1 Fill each pitta bread generously with an assortment of grated vegetables lightly moistened with a Super Salad Dressing (pages 44–46) or a dip from the Life of the Party (pages 63–65).

2 Arrange decoratively, alternating the colours, and garnish with sprigs of parsley or coriander. Serve with soup, salad, or a vegetable dish for lunch or dinner, or alone for tea, and with crudités for cocktail parties.

Soups for the Hungry

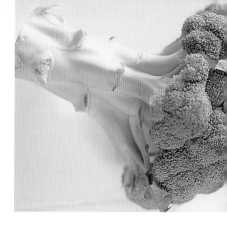

Miracle Vegetable Soup

per portion: 124 kcals • 4 g protein • 1 g fat • 25 g CHO

Serves 8

6 large onions

2 x 400 g (4 oz) cans peeled tomatoes

1 large white cabbage

2 green peppers

2 packets onion soup

1 celery stick

4 carrots, diced

pepper

1 dried bay leaf

1 Chop all the vegetables.

2 Place all the ingredients in a large saucepan and add just enough water to cover. Bring to the boil and simmer for 1 hour.

3 Store for up to 1 week.

(Note: This soup can be a starter, a snack or an entire meal! To lose weight really rapidly, just eat this soup for lunch and dinner every day for 1 week. You will always feel satisfied, and your reward will be a much trimmer body.)

Pennsylvania Mushroom Soup

per portion: 43 kcals • 3 g protein • 0 g fat • 4 g CHO

Serves 6

1 small onion, finely chopped

450 g (1 lb) mushrooms, finely chopped

1.1 litres (2 pints) chicken stock

2 tbs flour

pinch of salt and freshly ground black pepper

pinch of grated nutmeg

1 dried bay leaf

fresh parsley, to garnish

1 Add the onion and mushrooms to 2 tablespoons of chicken stock. Cover and cook gently for 5 minutes over medium heat.

2 Stir in the flour and continue cooking for 2 minutes, stirring constantly.

3 Gradually add the remaining chicken stock and bring to a boil, stirring. Add salt, pepper, nutmeg and bay leaf.

4 Lower the heat, half-cover, and simmer gently for 20 minutes.

Before serving, remove the bay leaf. Top each bowl of soup with a sprig of parsley.

Green Dream Broccoli Soup

per portion: 24 kcals • 2 g protein • 0 g fat • 4 g CHO

Serves 5

1 onion, sliced

1 carrot, sliced

1 small celery stick with leaves, sliced

1 garlic clove

120 ml (4 fl oz) water

120 g (4 oz) broccoli, cooked and coarsely chopped

1 tsp salt

pinch of cayenne pepper

25 g (1 oz) cooked macaroni

225 ml (8 fl oz) chicken stock

5 small florets of broccoli, steamed, to garnish

1 Bring the water to the boil, reduce the heat and add the onion, carrot, celery and garlic. Cover and simmer for 10 minutes.

2 Transfer to a blender. Add the broccoli, salt, cayenne pepper and macaroni. Cover and blend on high. With motor running, add the chicken stock and blend until the mixture is creamy.

3 Chill, and serve. Top each bowl with a floret of broccoli.

Tomato Basilique

per portion: 70 kcals • 5 g protein • 1 g fat • 12 g CHO

Cucumber Cooler

per portion: 26 kcals • 1 g protein • 0 g fat • 5 g CHO

Serves 6

3 cucumbers, peeled and deseeded

700 ml (1¼ pints) chicken stock

1 leek, white section only

1 dried bay leaf, crumbled

1 tbs plain flour

1 tbs lemon juice

4 tsp fresh dill or mint, chopped

freshly ground black pepper

1 In a saucepan sauté 2 cucumbers gently in 50 ml (2 fl oz) chicken stock with the leek and bay leaf for 20 minutes, or until tender but not browned.

2 Stir in the flour.

3 Add the remaining chicken stock and simmer for 30 minutes.

4 Put the mixture through a food mill or blend (half at a time); strain through a fine sieve. Chill.

5 Stir 1 grated cucumber into the mixture with the dill or mint. Add pepper to taste.

6 Chill for at least 2 hours. Serve cold in pre-chilled cups or reheat and serve hot.

Serves 4

1 x 400 g (14 oz) can whole Italian plum tomatoes, undrained

50 g (2 oz) chopped onion

1 tbs dried basil or 1 tsp finely chopped fresh basil

1 garlic clove

¼ tsp salt

¼ tsp white pepper

½ tsp low-fat margarine

1 tbs plus 1½ tsp plain flour

350 ml (12 fl oz) skimmed milk

To garnish:

50 g (2 oz) tomatoes, peeled and chopped

4 small leaves fresh basil

1 Place canned tomatoes, onion, basil, garlic, salt and pepper in a medium saucepan and bring to a boil. Cover, reduce heat and simmer for 10 minutes.

2 Place the mixture in a blender and process until smooth.

3 Melt the margarine in a small saucepan over low heat. Add the flour, stirring until smooth. Cook for 1 minute, stirring constantly.

4 Add the milk gradually. Cook over a low heat, stirring constantly, until thickened and bubbly.

5 Add the milk mixture to the tomato mixture, stirring. Heat for several minutes, stirring until thickened.

6 Garnish each bowl of soup with the chopped tomatoes and fresh basil.

Red Cabbage and Apple Soup

per portion: 37 kcals • 2 g protein • 0 g fat • 8 g CHO

Serves 8

1 leek, chopped

1 garlic clove, crushed

1 litre (1¾ pints) water

340 g (12 oz) red cabbage, shredded

120 ml (4 fl oz) tomato juice

1 tsp Worcestershire sauce

1 apple, chopped

1 potato, chopped

1 large chicken stock cube, crumbled

1 tbs chopped fresh chives, to garnish

1 In a non-stick saucepan, cook the leek and garlic in 50 ml (2 fl oz) water over medium heat for about 10 minutes (or microwave on HIGH for about 5 minutes) or until the leek is tender.

2 Add the cabbage, tomato juice, Worcestershire sauce, apple, potato, remaining water and stock cube. Bring to a boil, then reduce the heat, cover, and simmer for 30 minutes (or microwave on HIGH for 15 minutes) or until the potato is tender.

3 Blend the mixture in batches until smooth. Reheat gently; do not boil. Garnish with chives.

The Great Gazpacho

per portion: 34 kcals • 1 g protein • 1 g fat • 5 g CHO

Serves 6

1 large onion, preferably a red Spanish onion

2 garlic cloves, mashed

5 large, ripe tomatoes, peeled and diced

20 g (¾ oz) freshly chopped parsley

1 large green pepper, deseeded (optional)

2 cucumbers peeled (optional)

120 g (4 oz) celery, diced (optional)

¼ tsp paprika

2 tbs vinegar

2 tsp olive oil

225 ml (8 fl oz) light, low-salt chicken broth

2 drops Tabasco sauce (optional)

1 Liquidize the onion and garlic together in a blender.

2 Chop together the tomatoes and pepper, cucumber, and celery.

3 Mix the remaining ingredients together in a blender with the onion and garlic for 2 minutes. Season with Tabasco sauce if liked.

4 Chill for at least 4 hours.

5 Serve in chilled dishes. Pass round the finely chopped vegetables (green peppers, cucumbers, celery, peeled tomatoes, pimentos) and cubes of toasted low-calorie bread to be sprinkled on top separately.

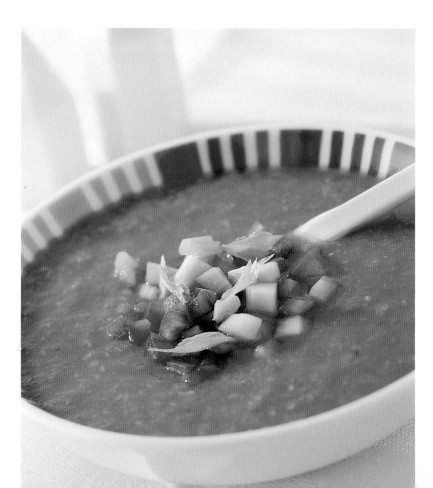

Pop-eye Potage

per portion: 65 kcals • 4 g protein • 2 g fat • 9 g CHO

Serves 6

600 g (1¼ lb) fresh spinach

15 g (½ oz) low-calorie margarine

1 onion, chopped

600 ml (1 pint) chicken stock

2 tbs flour

pinch of salt

freshly ground black pepper

freshly grated nutmeg (optional)

low-fat yogurt

6 slices of lemon

1 Wash the spinach thoroughly. Do not drain; put directly into a saucepan. (The water from the wet spinach is sufficient for cooking it.) Stir over medium heat, turning frequently, for 4 minutes, until soft. Add the margarine.

2 Transfer the cooked spinach to a blender, and purée slowly until smooth.

3 In another pan, cook the onion in a few tablespoons of stock; do not brown. Add the flour and cook for 3 minutes.

4 Mix the spinach into the onion. Bring to a boil, reduce the heat and simmer for 5 minutes. Cool.

5 Pour the mixture into the blender and purée until smooth.

6 Return the mixture to the saucepan and add sufficient stock for the soup to reach desired consistency. Add salt and pepper to taste.

7 To serve, reheat gently, but do not boil. Garnish each bowl with nutmeg, if liked, a dollop of low-fat yogurt and a slice of lemon.

Watercress Delight

per portion: 83 kcals • 5 g protein • 1 g fat • 16 g CHO

Serves 4

1 small onion, finely chopped

2 bunches of watercress, finely chopped

225 g (8 oz) potatoes, peeled and diced (½ to 1 potato)

340 ml (12 fl oz) chicken stock

340 ml (12 fl oz) skimmed milk

pinch of salt and freshly ground black pepper

few watercress leaves, to garnish

1 Put the vegetables in a saucepan with 3 tbs of chicken stock. Cover and cook for 5 minutes.

2 Stir in the milk and the remaining chicken stock and bring to a boil. Lower the heat, half-cover, and simmer gently for 30 minutes, stirring occasionally. Season.

3 Transfer the soup to a blender and purée. Return the soup to the rinsed-out pan and reheat.

4 Garnish each soup bowl with a few leaves of watercress.

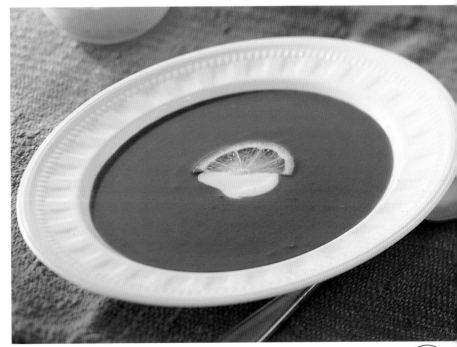

Super Salads

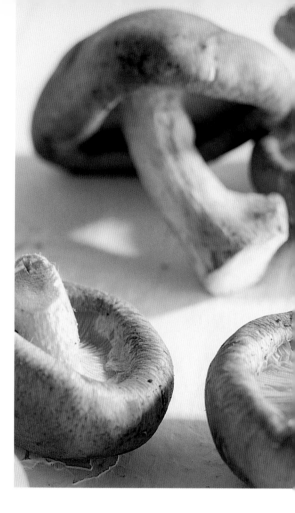

Salads are the most important foods for attaining and maintaining a cellulite-free body. Low in kilocalories and fat, high in fibre, rich with vitamins and minerals, salads are very healthy. And they demonstrate the greatest variety of any food: salads can be elegant starters, side dishes, snacks, or entire meals for lunch or dinner. You get the pleasure of munching, and you may eat as much as you want!

There is a whole wonderful world of salads. Made to suit any taste, salads can be dramatic dishes that make a strong impression when brought to the table. Dazzle your family and impress your guests! With salads, staying healthy and thin doesn't need to be dull. The variety of salads has no limits except your own imagination. And salads are great on the budget, too.

Salads are easy to make. You can always keep washed lettuce, spinach and chicory stored in the refrigerator covered with damp kitchen paper. Crudités can be cut and stored in the refrigerator propped in a container with a little water to keep them fresh and crunchy. You can make large quantities of salad dressing recipes and refrigerate them for up to two months.

The trick of the satisfying salad is to mix lots of fresh Fibre Feast vegetable ingredients and to add just a little dressing to enhance the flavour and make the salad satisfying and filling. Varying the dressing and the vegetable and fruit ingredients from day to day makes each salad a new and exciting treat!

Chicory Salad

per portion: 18 kcals • 0.5 g protein • 2 g fat • 0.5 g CHO

Serves 4

Wash about 2 chicory heads and cut into bite-sized slices. Combine with 1 bunch of watercress leaves, chopped. Add 1 tablespoon of Oil-free Vinaigrette (page 44). Place the portions directly on salad plates for an elegant first course or for a side salad.

Spinach Salad

per portion: 30 kcals • 5 g protein • 3 g CHO

Serves 4

450 g (1 lb) spinach, freshly washed

120 g (4 oz), freshly chopped

120 g (4 oz) sliced mushrooms

2 hard-boiled egg yolks, diced

4 hard-boiled egg whites, diced

½ red or yellow pepper, cut into thin slices

1 Remove stems of spinach and tear into bite-sized pieces.

2 Mix together chicory, mushrooms, eggs and pepper slivers. Toss into spinach.

3 Add salad dressing and toss.

(Note: For a special treat, preheat the salad dressing.)

Creative Horizon Salad

per portion: 100 kcals • 9 g protein • 2 g fat • 12 g CHO

Add to the lettuce any combination of:

chopped red onions and/or spring onions

sliced green, red or yellow peppers

grated courgettes

sliced mushrooms

diced celery

coriander

wedges of tomato

hearts of palm

canned artichoke

small chunks of turkey or chicken

tiny cubes of goat's cheese

egg whites

raisins

grapes

orange sections

pineapple

apple cubes (pre-soaked in lemon juice)

There are many tasty varieties of lettuce such as iceberg, cos, lollo rosso, butterhead and rocket, as well as salad greens such as chicory, spinach, and cabbage. Choose the type you most prefer or mix two or three kinds for a super mixed green salad.

Toss together with salad dressing. Garnish with tomatoes, onion rings, yellow, red or green pepper, celery, canned artichokes and/or apple cubes, coriander, parsley, orange slivers, grapes or pineapple sections.

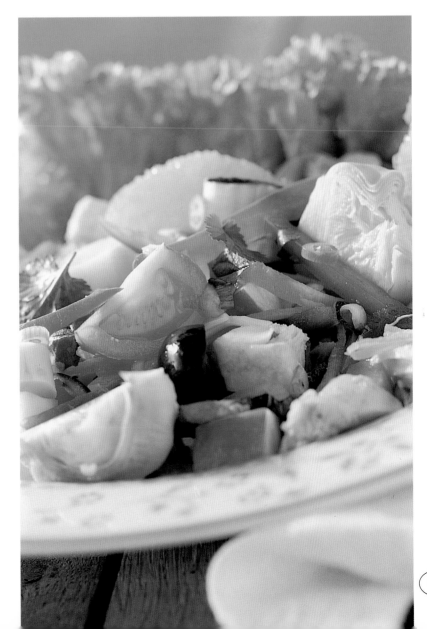

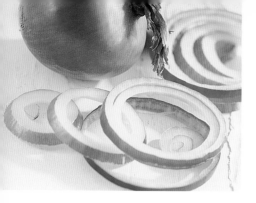

Bean Trio

per portion: 45 kcals • 4 g protein
• 0 g fat • 5 g CHO

Serves 4

Mix together 175 g (6 oz) each of lightly steamed green beans, yellow runner beans, and broad beans, 1 sliced raw red onion, and parsley to taste. Add 1 tablespoon Oil-free Vinaigrette (page 44). Marinate for 1 hour.

(Note: This salad is high in carbohydrate, so preferably should not be eaten with protein.)

Gazpacho Aspic

per portion: 38 kcals • 2 g protein
• 1 g fat • 4 g CHO

Serves 6

This is a variation of The Great Gazpacho (page 38). Soften 2 tablespoons of unflavoured gelatine in room-temperature water, then dissolve by heating it gently in the chicken stock. Do not boil. Chill the stock slightly before adding the other ingredients. Chill for at least 5 hours in moulds or cups. Turn out and serve on a bed of lettuce. Hand round separate bowls of chopped vegetables.

Cauliflower Italiano

per portion: 18 kcals • 1 g protein
• 0 g fat • 2.4 g CHO

Serves 8

200 g (7 oz) cauliflower florets, thinly sliced

25 g (1 oz) red pepper, chopped

25 g (1 oz) celery, sliced

1 tbs chopped spring onion

50 ml (2 oz) plain low-fat yogurt

3 tbs low-calorie Italian salad dressing

8 leaves red leaf lettuce

1 Combine the cauliflower, red pepper, celery and spring onion in a bowl.

2 Combine the yogurt and salad dressing. Pour over the vegetable mixture and toss.

3 Spoon the mixture evenly over lettuce leaves for individual servings.

Tuna Waldorf Salad

per portion: 48 kcals • 8 g protein
• 0 g fat • 4 g CHO

Serves 5

1 green or red apple, unpeeled

1 tbs lemon juice

150 g (4 oz) water-packed canned tuna fish, drained and flaked

1 tbs chopped pickle

1 tbs chopped pimento

20 g (¾ oz) raw Chinese cabbage or 50 g (2 oz) cucumber, chopped

85 g (3 oz) celery, finely chopped

lettuce, to serve

To garnish:

green beans, cooked and chopped

celery, diced

radishes, diced

pimento and/or tomato

1 Core, but do not peel, the apple, grate and sprinkle with lemon juice.

2 Mix with all of the remaining ingredients and chill.

3 Serve on a bed of lettuce.

4 Garnish with chopped cooked green beans, diced raw celery, diced radishes, pimento and/or tomato.

Key West Crab Salad

per portion: 145 kcals • 26 g protein • 4 g fat
• 9 g CHO

Serves 4

450 g (1 lb) lump crab meat

125 g (4 oz) heart of celery, finely chopped

40 g (1½ oz) spring onions, finely chopped

20 g (¾ oz) fresh parsley, finely chopped

Nancy's Vinaigrette Citron (page 44)

lettuce, to serve

To garnish:

*4 large fresh tomatoes, at least 7.5 cm
(3 inches) in diameter. Beefsteak tomatoes are
the best since they have the fewest seeds.*

16 pieces canned artichoke

1 Wash and drain the crab meat.

2 Mix the heart of celery, spring onions and
fresh parsley with crab meat in a bowl. Chill.

3 Add 4 tablespoons of Nancy's Vinaigrette
Citron (page 44). Mix thoroughly.

4 Serve on lettuce, garnish with tomatoes and
artichoke pieces, and sprinkle with Nancy's
Vinaigrette Citron.

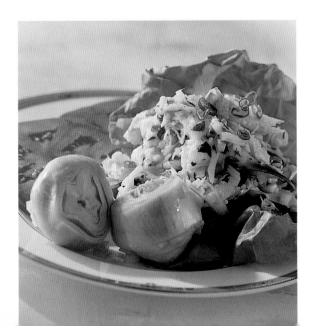

Cumberland Salad

per portion: 153 kcals • 4 g protein • 4 g fat
• 26 g CHO

Serves 4

125 g (4 oz) pearl barley

350 ml (12 fl oz) stock or water

125 g (4 oz) broccoli florets, lightly cooked

1 celery stick, finely chopped

1 small carrot, shredded

4 tbs balsamic or sherry wine vinegar

1 tbs olive oil

2 tbs Pommeray mustard or herb mustard

2 tbs chopped fresh basil

2 tbs water

pinch of salt and freshly ground black pepper

lettuce, to serve

fresh basil, to garnish

1 Place the pearl barley and stock or water in
a saucepan and bring to a boil. Reduce heat
to medium and cook for 45 minutes or until
slightly soft. Rinse under cold water and drain.

2 Mix the barley with the vegetables.

3 In a bowl combine the vinegar, olive oil,
mustard, basil and salt and pepper. Mix into
the barley and vegetables.

4 Allow the salad to marinate for 20 minutes
before serving. Serve on a bed of lettuce and
garnish with fresh basil.

(Note: This is a hearty, filling salad which is
high in carbohydrate and, ideally, should not
be eaten with protein.)

Dressing It Up

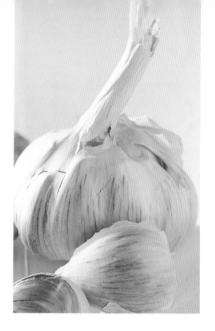

Oil-Free Vinaigrette

per tablespoon: 7 kcals • 0 g fat
• 0 g protein • 0 g CHO

Makes 240 ml (8 fl oz)

120 ml (4 fl oz) white wine

120 ml (4 fl oz) your favourite vinegar

3 tbs strong Dijon mustard

1 tbs chopped fresh sage or ½ tsp dried sage

1 tbs chopped shallots

salt and freshly ground black pepper

Put all of the ingredients into a screw-top jar. Close tightly and shake well.

(Note: This vinaigrette is easy to prepare and very tasty. It keeps in the refrigerator for as long as a month; just shake it well before using it. You can vary the taste by using different vinegars and by adding fresh or dried herbs; and you can even combine herbs if you choose. Best of all, this dressing contains no fat!)

Nancy's Vinaigrette Citron

per tablespoon: 9 kcals
• 0 g protein • 1 g fat • 0 g CHO

Makes 225 ml (8 fl oz)

10 tbs lemon juice

1 tbs olive oil

1 tsp white pepper

1 tsp Dijon mustard

4 tbs balsamic vinegar

1 tbs finely chopped garlic

Put all of the ingredients into a small screw-top jar. Close tightly and shake well. Let stand for 12 minutes.

(Note: This dressing must be added to the salad just before eating.)

Dijon Vinaigrette

per tablespoon: 22 kcals
• 0 g protein • 2.5 g fat • 0 g CHO

Makes about 4 tablespoons

⅛ tsp salt

¼ tsp black pepper

1 tbs Dijon mustard

2 tbs red wine vinegar

1 tbs olive oil

Put all of the ingredients into a small screw-top jar. Close tightly and shake well.

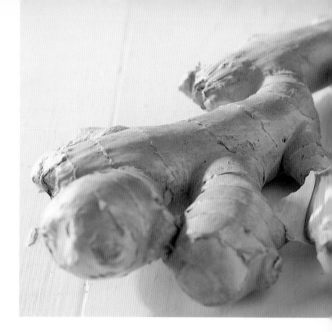

Herb Ginger Vinaigrette

per tablespoon: 11 kcals
• 0 g protein • 2 g fat• 0 g CHO

Makes 120 ml (4 fl oz)

5 cm (2 in) cube fresh ginger, grated

1 bunch chervil, washed and patted dry, leaves and tops of stems only, chopped

1 tbs olive oil

4 tbs rice wine vinegar

2 tbs lemon juice

1 tsp Dijon mustard

1 tsp chopped parsley

1 tsp chopped shallot

⅛ tsp salt

¼ tsp freshly ground black pepper

Put all of the ingredients into a small screw-top jar. Close tightly and shake well.

Tart Vinaigrette

per tablespoon: 145 kcals
• 0 g protein • 2 g fat • 0 g CHO

Makes 175 ml (6 fl oz)

2 tbs extra virgin olive oil

150 ml (5½ fl oz) red wine vinegar

1 garlic clove, crushed

½ tsp dried oregano

1 anchovy, finely chopped or puréed in a blender (optional)

black pepper, to taste

Put all of the ingredients into a small screw-top jar. Close tightly and shake well.

Sesame Salad Dressing

per tablespoon: 15 kcals
• 0 g protein • 1 g fat • 0 g CHO

Makes 600 ml (1 pint)

60 ml (2 fl oz) dark sesame oil

300 ml (10 fl oz) red wine vinegar

180 ml (6 fl oz) water

120 ml (4 fl oz) low-sodium soy sauce

Put all of the ingredients into a small screw-top jar. Close tightly and shake well. Store in the refrigerator for up to 1 month.

(Note: This dressing goes especially well with spinach and crudités. It can also be used with grilled fish and poultry.)

Anchovy French Dressing

per tablespoon: 32 kcals
• 2 g protein • 2.5 g fat • 0 g CHO

Makes about 7 tablespoons

50 g (2 oz) anchovy fillets

1 tbs olive oil

4 tbs lemon juice

1 spring onion (optional)

Drain the anchovies and pat dry on kitchen paper. Cut them into tiny pieces. Put all of the ingredients into a small screw-top jar. Close tightly and shake well.

Mayo-n-eze

per level tablespoon: 40 kcals
• 0 g protein • 5 g fat • 0 g CHO

Makes about 14 tablespoons

1 egg

½ tsp dry mustard

4 tbs olive oil

4 tbs apple cider vinegar or lemon juice

seasonings (see below)

Put the ingredients in a blender and mix at high speed. If the mixture gets very thick, stop the blender and stir with a spatula before continuing to blend. Season with pepper, grated onion or onion powder, garlic or dill.

African Lemon Dressing

per tablespoon: 28 kcals
• 0 g protein • 3 g fat • 0.5 g CHO

Makes about 8 tablespoons

rind of 2 lemons, grated

4 tbs lemon juice

¼ tsp salt

⅛ tsp white pepper

2 garlic cloves finely chopped

2 tbs olive oil

½ tsp ground coriander

1 tsp ground cumin

1 tsp Dijon mustard

1½ tsp artificial sweetener

½ tsp paprika

Put all of the ingredients into a small screw-top jar. Close tightly and shake well.

Herb Sauce

per tablespoon: 1.6 kcals
• 0 g protein • 0 g fat • 0 g CHO

Makes about 10 tablespoons

120 ml (4 fl oz) lemon juice

4 tbs balsamic vinegar

⅛ tsp powdered thyme

⅛ tsp powdered marjoram

1½ tsp dried basil

4 fresh basil leaves, chopped

1 tbs water

¼ tsp salt

5 tbs fresh chopped parsley

Put all of the ingredients into a small screw-top jar. Close tightly and shake well. Let stand for 12 minutes.

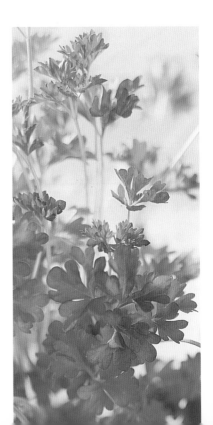

Starting Right

Starters were created to stimulate the appetite, but when they are chosen properly, they can also satisfy it.

All of the recipes given here are satisfying, tasty, easy to prepare, low in kilocalories, and healthy. They are elegant enough to serve to guests and they can also stand alone as the main course of a light luncheon.

The Soups for the Hungry (pages 36–39) and Super Salads (pages 40–43) also make excellent starters!

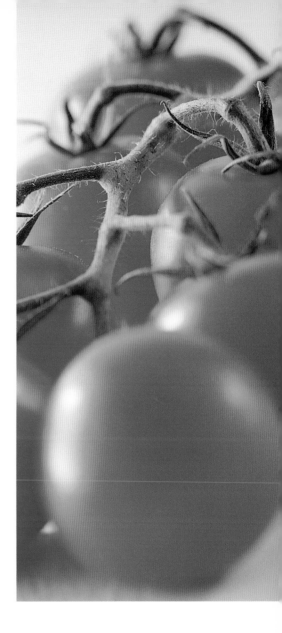

Tomatoes Provençal

per portion: 30 kcals • 1.5 g protein • 0 g fat • 7 g CHO

Serves 2

2 large tomatoes or 10 large cherry tomatoes

2 tbs crushed garlic

2 spring onions, cut into ringlets

4 tbs fat-free chicken stock

1 tsp white pepper

1 tsp dried oregano

2 large courgettes, grated with skin

5 tbs chopped parsley

fresh parsley, to garnish

1 Cut the large tomatoes in half and remove the seeds. If using cherry tomatoes, remove the stems and cut the tops off, put the tops aside and scoop out the seeds with a small spoon.

2 Brown the garlic and onion in 2 tablespoons of stock and season.

3 Add the courgette, parsley and the rest of the chicken stock. Heat for a few minutes until the courgette is just soft.

4 Drain the cooked vegetables on kitchen paper. Spoon them into the tomato shells; replace the tops of the cherry tomatoes. Garnish with fresh parsley.

Gourmet Goat's Cheese Soufflé

per portion: 134 kcals • 9 g protein • 7 g fat • 12 g CHO

Serves 10

2 tbs low-calorie unsalted margarine

4 tbs fresh breadcrumbs

3 tbs plain flour

350 ml (12 fl oz) skimmed milk

225 g (8 oz) soft mild goat's cheese, such as Montrachet, crumbled

3 large egg yolks

7 large egg whites

salt and pepper, to taste

lettuce, to serve

1 Preheat oven to 190° C (375°F), Gas Mark 5. Wipe 8 x 120 ml (4 oz) ramekins sparingly with margarine and coat well with breadcrumbs, knocking out excess and reserving for sprinkling soufflés.

2 In a medium saucepan, melt the margarine over low heat and whisk in the flour. Cook for 3 minutes, stirring constantly.

3 Stir in milk, and bring to a boil. Remove from the heat.

4 In a large bowl, mix together 175 g (6 oz) of the cheese, egg yolks, salt and pepper. Add to the flour and milk in the saucepan and cook just to boiling point.

5 Beat the egg whites until they just hold stiff peaks.

6 Fold the egg whites carefully and thoroughly into the cheese mixture.

7 Divide the mixture equally between the ramekins.

8 Place the ramekins in a roasting tin. Add enough hot water to roasting tin to go halfway up the sides of the ramekins. Bake soufflés in the middle of the oven for about 25 minutes, until golden brown. Remove pan from oven and let stand in the tin for 15 minutes.

9 Run a knife around the edge of each soufflé and turn out on to a baking sheet. The soufflés may be prepared up to this point 1½ hours ahead of time and kept at room temperature.

10 Preheat the oven to 220°C (425°F), Gas Mark 7. Bake the soufflés on a baking sheet in the middle of the oven until puffed and golden brown, about 5–7 minutes.

11 Serve on lettuce lightly moistened with the vinaigrette of your choice.

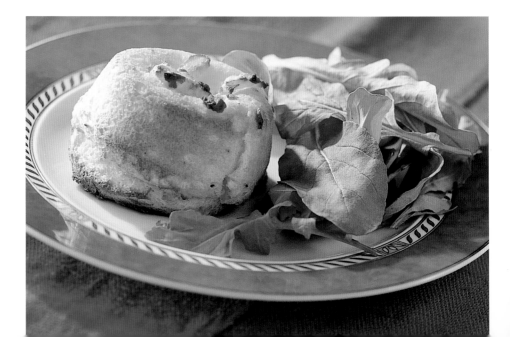

Light Chicken Terrine

per portion: 177 kcals • 23 g protein • 5 g fat • 10 g CHO

Serves 8

1 red pepper, deseeded and chopped

1 green pepper, deseeded and chopped

120 g (4 oz) carrots, diced

50 g (2 oz) onion, diced

600 g (1¼ lb) boneless chicken breasts, skinned

1 tsp chicken-flavoured stock granules

½ tsp white pepper

½ tsp curry powder

½ tsp hot sauce

370 ml (13 fl oz) skimmed milk

4 tbs dry white wine

1 egg

1 egg white

1 bunch cos lettuce

To garnish:

slivers of green or red pepper

1 Steam the peppers, carrots and onion over boiling water for 10 minutes. Drain and set aside.

2 Cut chicken into 2.5 cm (1 inch) pieces. Put half of it into a blender with the stock granules, pepper, curry powder and hot sauce. Blend until smooth, scraping the blender once. Slowly add 175 ml (6 fl oz) evaporated milk, the wine and egg, blending until smooth. Pour into a large bowl.

3 Blend the rest of the chicken with the remaining evaporated milk and the egg white. Stir the two chicken mixtures together.

4 Line the bottom and sides of a non-stick loaf tin with the lettuce leaves (dull side up). Allow the leaves to hang over sides of the tin.

5 Spread half of the chicken mixture into the tin. Spoon the steamed vegetables on top of the chicken, then spread the remaining chicken over the vegetables.

6 Cover the tin tightly with aluminium foil, punching a hole in the foil for steam to escape. Place loaf tin in a roasting tin. Fill the roasting tin with hot water to a depth of 3.5 cm (1½ inches).

7 Bake at 180°C (350°F), Gas Mark 4 for 1¼ hours or until the terrine is firm and the centre springs back after touching. Remove the foil from loaf tin and allow to cool. When warm to the touch, pour off the excess liquid. Cool completely.

8 Turn out the terrine on to a serving dish. Cover with clingfilm and refrigerate overnight.

9 Let stand at room temperature 30 minutes before serving. Garnish with slivers of green or red pepper.

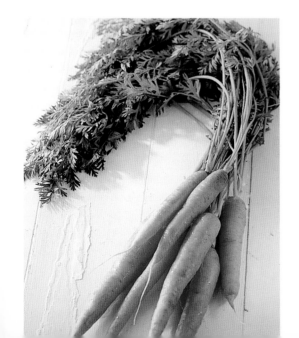

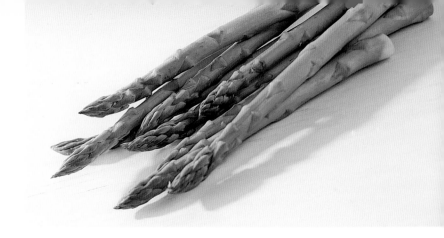

Magic Mushrooms

per portion: 33 kcals
- 2 g protein • 1 g fat • 5 g CHO

Serves 6

225 g (8 oz) shiitake mushrooms

225 g (8 oz) oyster mushrooms

225 g (8 oz) snow mushrooms

1 tsp dried oregano

1 tsp rosemary

1 tsp thyme

8 tbs chopped parsley

3 shallots, well chopped

1 tsp olive oil

juice of 2 limes

¼ tsp pepper

lettuce greens of choice

1 Remove stems from mushrooms. Wipe each mushroom gently with a damp paper towel.

2 Chop all herbs together.

3 Mix olive oil and lime juice; then add pepper and herbs.

4 Marinate mushrooms and shallots in the seasoned oil/lime mixture for 2–3 hours at room temperature (the longer the better).

5 Drain the mushrooms and shallots and sauté in a non-stick frying pan for about 5 minutes, turning frequently. Alternatively, heat in the oven at 200°C (400°F), Gas Mark 6 for 15 minutes, stirring several times.

6 Serve warm on the greens of your choice.

Fresh Asparagus Premier

per portion: 35 kcals • 9 g protein
- 0 g fat • 5 g CHO

Serves 2

450 g (1 lb) asparagus

225 ml (8 fl oz) water

salt and pepper, to taste

hard-boiled egg whites, to garnish

1 Wash the asparagus well. Trim the hard root ends from the stalk, then pare away the tough skin using a potato peeler.

2 Fresh asparagus is best cooked by standing upright in a deep pan so that the delicate tips are gently softened. Alternatively, the asparagus can be laid flat in a frying pan, preferably with a steamer tray.

3 Steam asparagus, covered, until tender when pierced with a fork (about 8–12 minutes). Drain and save the liquid as stock.

4 Serve the asparagus hot or chilled, topped with the vinaigrette of your choice (pages 44–45) and garnished with grated hard-boiled egg whites.

Artichokes Royale

per portion: 37 kcals • 2 g protein
- 0 g fat • 6 g CHO

1 artichoke per person

lemon juice

pinch sea salt

2 cloves garlic (optional)

lemon slice, to garnish

1 Trim the artichoke stalks and remove the leaves around the base. Rub the artichoke with lemon juice to prevent discoloration.

2 Place the artichokes in salted boiling water; cook over low heat for about 40 minutes. If you wish, flavour the water with diced garlic.

3 Serve hot or cold with the vinaigrette of your choice (see pages 44–45). Garnish with a slice of lemon.

The Main Event

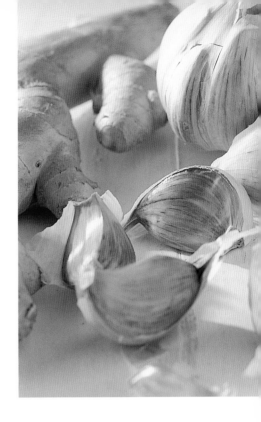

The main courses that follow are easy to prepare, low in kcals and fat, and absolutely delicious and elegant. No one will believe that these delicious meals are really healthy!

Chicken is lower in fat and kilocalories than other meats, and turkey is even lower. A portion is 75 g (3 oz). All of the chicken recipes can be made with turkey instead. A great method for cooking fowl or fish is *en papillote*. Place the chicken or fish on a piece of baking parchment, add herbs and lemon juice (and a dab of tomato sauce, if you wish), fold and bake at 180°C (350°F), Gas Mark 4 for 40 minutes. The parchment seals in the juices.

A quick, lively, and unusual sauce for chicken or fish can be made with a purée of 3 red peppers blended with 3 tablespoons of chicken stock.

Sunny Chicken

per portion: 184 kcals • 25 g protein • 5 g fat • 11 g CHO

Serves 4

450 g (1 lb) boneless raw chicken

120 ml (4 fl oz) orange juice

4 tbs soy sauce

4 tbs ketchup

1 tbs honey

1 tsp salt

1 tsp fresh basil leaves

¼ tsp pepper

1 Place the chicken in a large shallow baking dish.

2 In a bowl, combine the orange juice, soy sauce, ketchup, honey, salt, basil and pepper. Pour over the chicken.

3 Bake uncovered at 180°C (350°F), Gas Mark 4 for 1 hour or until done.

Herb Cognac Chicken

per portion: 187 kcals • 24 g protein • 4 g fat • 2 g CHO

Serves 4

1 boned and skinned chicken, cut into bite-sized pieces

4 tbs chicken broth

2 garlic cloves, crushed

225 ml (8 fl oz) dry white wine

2 tbs cognac

2 tbs low-calorie tomato purée

1 tsp salt

1 tsp dried thyme

1 Brown the chicken pieces in a non-stick frying pan. Add the broth and baste the chicken to moisten.

2 In a bowl, mix together the garlic, wine, cognac, tomato purée, salt and thyme. Add mixture to the chicken.

3 Cover and simmer for 30 minutes or until done.

Tangy Barbecued Chicken

per portion: 135 kcals • 20 g protein • 3 g fat • 7 g CHO

Serves 4

450 g (1 lb) boned and skinned chicken breast halves

4 tbs reduced sodium ketchup

3 tbs cider vinegar

1 tbs ready-made white horseradish

2 tsp dark brown sugar

1 garlic clove, finely chopped

¼ tsp dried thyme

¼ tsp black pepper

1 Heat a charcoal grill until coals form white ash, or preheat a grill to medium.

2 In a small saucepan, combine the ketchup, vinegar, horseradish, brown sugar, garlic and thyme. Mix well and bring to a boil over medium-low heat. Cook, stirring frequently, until thickened, about 5 minutes. Remove from the heat; stir in the pepper.

3 Brush the tops of chicken pieces lightly with sauce. Place the chicken, sauce-side down, on a grill rack. Brush the other sides lightly with sauce.

4 Grill 7.5 cm (3 inches) from the heat, basting with remaining sauce and turning until no longer pink in the centre, about 5–7 minutes a side. Let the chicken stand for 5 minutes before serving.

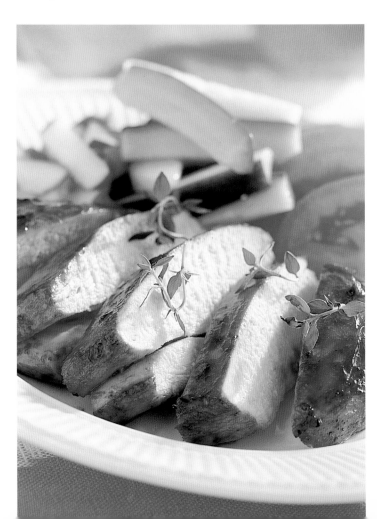

Spinach Roulade Sole

per portion: 143 kcals • 21 g protein • 2 g fat
• 13 g CHO

Serves 4

4 tbs lemon juice

½ tsp onion powder

1 garlic clove, chopped

4 x 85 g (3 oz) pieces of sole (lemon sole, Dover sole or flounder)

900 g (2 lb) fresh spinach, cut

125 ml (4 fl oz) chicken stock

4 slices red pepper

4 tsp dried breadcrumbs

1 tbs fresh coriander, to garnish

1 Mix the lemon juice, onion powder and garlic.

2 Place the fish in a shallow dish, pour the lemon juice mixture on top, and marinate for 2 hours.

3 Cook the spinach in boiling chicken stock for 5 minutes. Drain and chop.

4 Remove the fish from the marinade and lay flat. Cover each piece with a quarter of the cooked spinach. Roll around 1 strip of red pepper and hold together with a cocktail stick.

5 Spray a baking dish with non-fat vegetable oil cooking spray. Place the fish in the dish. Top with coriander and 1 teaspoon of breadcrumbs per piece, to prevent dryness.

6 Bake at 200°C (400°F), Gas Mark 6 for 20–25 minutes.

Roast Monkfish with Red Wine Glaze

per portion: 146 kcals • 28 g protein • 1 g fat
• 7 g CHO

Serves 4

700 g (1½ lb) monkfish

2 garlic cloves, thinly sliced

2 tsp olive oil

1 tsp dried thyme

1 tbs frozen orange juice

½ tsp artificial sweetener

120 ml (4 fl oz) red wine

1 tbs red wine vinegar

1 tsp low-calorie tomato purée

1 tbs butter or low-fat margarine

1 Preheat the oven to 200°C (400°F), Gas Mark 6.

2 Trim the monkfish of all sinew. Cut little slits all over the monkfish and fill them with garlic. Place it in an ovenproof baking dish. Brush it with olive oil and sprinkle it with thyme.

3 Bake, uncovered, for 15 minutes or until white juices rise to the top.

4 Meanwhile combine the orange juice, sweetener, red wine, vinegar and tomato purée in a saucepan. Bring to a boil and cook until the liquid reduces to 75 ml (3 fl oz), about 3 minutes. Add in any accumulated juices from the monkfish and bring to a boil again.

5 Remove from the heat and whisk in the butter. The sauce should now be slightly thick and glossy.

6 Slice the monkfish into slices about 6 mm (¼ inch) thick and serve with a spoonful of the glaze.

Courgette Boats

per portion: 62 kcals • 5 g protein
• 4 g fat • 2.5 g CHO

Serves 8

8 courgettes, with skin

1 tbs olive oil

1 tsp chopped parsley

½ chopped onion

1 red pepper, chopped

2 tbs seasoned breadcrumbs

4 tsp grated Parmesan cheese (optional)

⅛ tsp salt

½ tsp white pepper

1 Preheat oven to 190°C (375°F), Gas Mark 5.

2 Cut the courgettes in half lengthways and scoop out pulp. Do not break the skin.

3 Heat the oil in a large frying pan over a low heat. Add the parsley and onion, and cook until the onion is light brown. Stir in the courgette pulp and chopped red pepper. Cook for 3 minutes.

4 Mix with the seasoned breadcrumbs, cheese, salt and pepper. Fill the courgettes with the mixture.

5 Place courgettes in a baking dish just large enough to hold them.

6 Bake for 20 minutes.

Coriander Swordfish

per portion: 178 kcals • 29 g protein
• 2 g fat • 0 g CHO

Serves 2

2 x 120 g (4 oz) pieces of swordfish (or pink salmon, lemon sole, Dover sole or flounder*)

4 tbs lemon juice

120 ml (4 fl oz) white wine

¼ tsp pepper

4 stems fresh coriander

To garnish:

lemon slices

coriander leaves

1 Marinate the fish in lemon juice and wine with pepper and coriander for 1–2 hours.

2 Place the fish in a baking dish spread with olive oil.

3 Grill for 10–12 minutes until brown.

4 Serve garnished with lemon slices and fresh coriander leaves.

*Sole and flounder have fewer kcals and less fat.

Vegetable Kebabs

per portion: 100 kcals • 4 g protein
• 3 g fat • 16 g CHO

Serves 6

1 aubergine, cut into chunks

36 small button mushrooms

1 red or green pepper, deseeded and cut into strips

24 pickling onions or 2 onions, cut into chunks

6 small courgettes, cut into thick slices

3 tbs Dijon mustard

3 garlic cloves, crushed

3 tbs dark brown sugar

3 tbs soy sauce

1 tbs olive oil

½ tsp salt

1 Sprinkle the aubergine with salt, let stand for 30 minutes, then rinse and drain.

2 Thread the vegetables on to 12 skewers. Lay the skewers flat on a non-metal tray or a large plate.

3 Mix together the mustard, garlic, brown sugar, soy sauce, olive oil and salt. Spoon the marinade over the vegetables, turning the skewers to coat all the vegetables. Marinate for at least 1 hour, basting occasionally.

4 Cook the kebabs on a barbecue or under a hot grill for 10–15 minutes, until tender.

5 Present the kebabs on a bed of Wholegrain Rice Bouquet (page 31). Serve the remaining marinade separately.

Nature's Vegetables

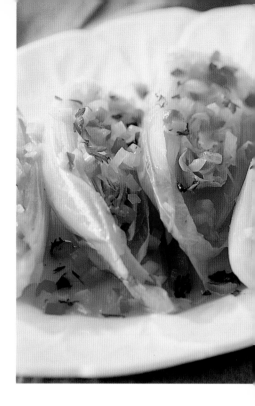

Vegetables are best when lightly steamed so they remain crunchy. This preserves not only the taste but also the valuable fibre and nutrients. Try different Fibre Feast vegetables such as fennel, okra, spaghetti squash, turnips and courgettes. Enhance the flavour with herbs and spices such as tarragon, caraway seeds, garlic, paprika, basil, marjoram, dill, thyme, parsley and oregano, and with balsamic vinegar or lemon juice. Do not add salt. For a true energy boost, drink the water remaining after steaming.

Choose the freshest vegetables, store in a cool, dark place and use within a couple of days. Frozen vegetables are good, too, because the best of the crop is chosen straight after picking for freezing, which preserves the nutrients.

String Beans Sesame

per portion: 40 kcals • 2 g protein • 1 g fat • 5 g CHO

Serves 4

680 g (1½ lb) string beans

2 tbs soy sauce

1 tbs Worcestershire sauce

2 tbs chicken stock

1 tbs sesame seed

⅛ tsp salt

½ tsp freshly ground black pepper

1 Wash stringbeans and trim ends.

2 Mix all other ingredients. Heat.

3 Add the string beans, cover and cook over a low heat for 4–6 minutes until tender.

Spinach Courgette Harmony

per portion: 27 kcals • 3 g protein • 1 g fat • 2 g CHO

Serves 6

1 courgette with skin

1 tsp olive oil

1 garlic clove, chopped

450 g (1 lb) spinach

120 ml (4 fl oz) chicken stock

1 Wash the courgette, scrubbing with a brush. Grate with a cheese grater.

2 Heat the olive oil with the garlic and sauté the courgette.

3 Cook the spinach in boiling chicken stock for 5 minutes. Mix with the courgette.

Spicy Chicory

per portion: 26 kcals • 1 g protein • 1 g fat • 6 g CHO

Serves 2

2 heads chicory (about 225 g/8 oz)

1 tbs celery, diced

1 tbs onion, chopped

1 tbs diced pimento

4 tbs water with 1 tbs lemon juice or chicken stock

¼ tsp chicken stock granules

1 Trim the chicory and remove any wilted leaves.

2 Cut the chicory in half lengthways. Place in a frying pan and sprinkle with celery, onion and pimento.

3 Combine water and lemon juice, or chicken stock, with the stock granules, stirring well. Pour over the chicory.

4 Bring to a boil. Cover, reduce heat, and simmer for 10 minutes.

Stock Fried Okra

per portion 23 kcals • 1 g protein • 0.5 g fat • 4 g CHO

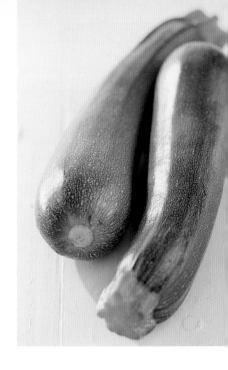

Serves 6

1 tbs chicken stock

225 g (8 oz) fresh okra, sliced or whole

50 g (2 oz) onion, chopped

1 red pepper, deseeded and diced

½ tsp whole basil

¼ tsp dried thyme

⅛ tsp pepper

1 tomato, chopped

1 In a large frying pan heat the chicken stock.

2 Add the sliced okra, onion, red pepper, basil, thyme and pepper. Stir-fry for 6 minutes or just until tender.

3 Add chopped tomato to mixture, and stir-fry for two minutes.

Mushrooms Sauté

per portion: 9 kcals • 1 g protein • 0 g fat • 1 g CHO

Serves 2

1 garlic clove, slightly crushed

4 tbs water

75 g (3 oz) mushrooms, thickly sliced

4 tbs lemon juice

1 Simmer the garlic in water in a non-stick frying pan for 5 minutes.

2 Remove the garlic and add the mushrooms and lemon juice.

3 Cook, stirring frequently, for 3–5 minutes or until mushrooms are tender.

Surprise Brussels Sprouts

per portion: 52 kcals • 4 g protein • 2 g fat • 6 g CHO

Serves 4

450 g (1 lb) fresh Brussels sprouts

½ tsp dried tarragon, crushed

4 tbs water

½-¾ red pepper, coarsely grated

2 tsp grated lemon rind

2 tbs lemon juice

1 Place Brussels sprouts, tarragon and water in a saucepan. Cover and bring to a boil.

2 Reduce heat, simmer for 8 minutes.

3 Add the red pepper. Cook 2 minutes or until just tender. Drain.

4 Sprinkle the lemon rind and juice over the vegetables and toss lightly.

Chablis Squash

per portion: 20 kcals • 1 g protein • 0 g fat • 3 g CHO

Serves 6

3 tbs Chablis or other dry white wine

1 small white onion, quartered and thinly sliced

2 courgettes, thinly sliced

2 yellow squash, thinly sliced

½ tsp chicken-flavoured stock granules

¼ tsp dried basil

⅛ tsp freshly ground black pepper

1 In a large frying pan, heat the wine.

2 Add the onion, and sauté for 1 minute.

3 Add the courgettes, yellow squash, and stock granules. Sauté for 3 minutes or until just tender.

4 Sprinkle with basil and pepper before serving.

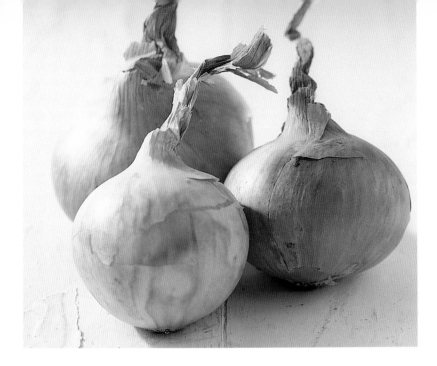

Rice Tricolore

per portion: 142 kcals • 3 g protein • 2 g fat • 31 g CHO

Serves 6

Rice:

200 g (7 oz) brown Basmati rice

570 ml (1 pint) water

1 onion, chopped

1 tsp olive oil

Tricolore:

50 g (2 oz) frozen peas, courgettes and/or spinach

85 g (3 oz) red peppers, diced

85 g (3 oz) yellow peppers, diced

1 Boil the rice in the water slowly with the onion and olive oil for 40–45 minutes until the water is fully absorbed.

2 Cook the frozen vegetables according to the instructions on the packet. Cut the spinach into large pieces. If using fresh courgette, grate and blanch in 1 tablespoon of water.

3 Blanch red and yellow peppers in 120 ml (4 fl oz) boiling water for a few seconds.

4 Mix the vegetables together with the rice as soon as they are cooked, while they are still hot.

(Note: This is a carbohydrate which should preferably be eaten with green salads and high-fibre vegetables and not with proteins.)

Cumin-Scented Spinach

per portion: 22 kcals • 3 g protein • 0 g fat • 2 g CHO

Serves 4

1 bunch of spinach, washed

1 tbs chicken stock

1 tsp ground cumin

1 tsp lime juice

pepper, to taste

1 Place the wet spinach in a saucepan. Cover and steam on medium heat until the spinach is just wilted, about 5 minutes.

2 Remove the spinach, drain it on kitchen paper to remove excess water. Cool to room temperature.

3 In the same saucepan, heat the chicken stock over medium heat. Stir in the cumin and spinach. Sauté until hot. Add the lime juice and pepper.

Caraway Cabbage

per portion: 15 kcals • 1 g protein • 0 g fat • 3 g CHO

Serves 4

120 g (4 oz) cabbage, thinly sliced

50 g (2 oz) celery, diced

50 g (2 oz) tomato, chopped

50 g (2 oz) red or green pepper, finely chopped

1 small onion, diced

1 tbs vinegar

¼ tsp caraway seeds

50 ml (2 fl oz) water

1 Combine all the ingredients in a large frying pan.

2 Cover and cook over a low heat for 6 minutes or until the vegetables are crisp but tender, stirring occasionally.

The Great Potato

per potato, approximately: 136 kcals • 4 g protein
• 0.2 g fat • 32 g CHO

1 Wash the potato thoroughly, using a small scrubbing brush if it is fresh from the soil.

2 With a paring knife, make an X in the centre top of the potato before baking (so that the potato does not explode!).

3 Bake in a preheated 200°C (400°F), Gas Mark 6 oven for 1 hour.

4 Split the potato in half. If using a white potato, remove most of the potato and save only the skin. Serve with tablespoons of one of the toppings below and garnish with a sprig of parsley. A sweet potato is delicious even without a topping!

(Note: An old-fashioned baked potato served with a delicious topping makes a hearty, filling and delightful breakfast or lunch. Since this is a carbohydrate, you should eat it with green salads and high fibre, green vegetables and not as a side dish with protein main courses. A whole potato has about 220 kcals, but if you eat the skin lined with just a bit of potato, there are only half the kcals with almost all of the nutrients. A sweet potato has only 118 kcals with an incredible number of nutrients including beta-carotene and the trace mineral selenium – both of which help prevent many forms of cancer. If you have a sweet tooth, a sweet potato is a fantastic meal – just like a dessert!)

Cheddar Cheese and Tomato Topping

per topping, using 25 g cheese:
68 kcals • 8 g protein • 4 g fat
• 0 g CHO

Top the slit potato with Cheddar cheese and a slice of tomato. Reheat it in the oven or under the grill for a few minutes, until the cheese melts.

Chive Topping

per tablespoon: 8 kcals
• 1 g protein • 0 g fat • 1 g CHO

Makes 16 tablespoons

Mix 225 ml (8 fl oz) very low-fat yogurt with 2 tablespoons of chives.

Parmesan Cheese Topping

per tablespoon: 14 kcals
• 1.5 g protein • 0 g fat • 1 g CHO

Makes 16 tablespoons

Mix 225 ml (8 fl oz) very low-fat yogurt with 2 tablespoons of grated Parmesan cheese.

Ricotta Cheese Topping

per tablespoon: 14 kcals
• 1 g protein • 1 g fat • 1 g CHO

Makes 16 tablespoons

Mix 120 g (4 oz) semi-skimmed ricotta cheese with 120 ml (4 fl oz) of very low-fat yogurt. This is especially delicious with a sweet potato. You can add ½ teaspoon of artificial sweetener if you like. For the non-sweet potato, you may enjoy seasoning with 3 tablespoons of chives.

Desserts: The Grand Finale

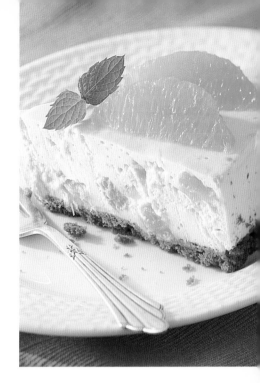

The very best dessert is fresh fruit! It can be presented with all the panache of a work of art. Sliced melon topped with lemon and a mint leaf, mixed berries, orange slices (sprinkled with Grand Marnier for special occasions), pineapple decorated with strawberries or raspberries – all satisfy your sweet tooth and end a meal with pizzazz. Here are some other great dessert recipes for you to try.

Orange Chiffon Cheese Cake

per portion: 159 kcals • 9 g protein • 7 g fat • 16 g CHO

Serves 12

150 g (5 oz) digestive biscuit crumbs

½ tsp cinnamon

50 g (2 oz) low-fat margarine, melted

225 ml (8 fl oz) fresh orange juice

2 tbs powdered gelatine

340 g (12 oz) low-calorie cream cheese, softened

225 g (8 oz) semi-skimmed ricotta cheese

3½ tsp artificial sweetener

1 packet low-calorie whipped topping mix

120 ml (4 fl oz) skimmed milk

2 oranges, peeled, deseeded and chopped

To decorate:

1 orange, peeled and segmented

mint leaves

1 Preheat the oven to 180°C (350°), Gas Mark 4.

2 Blend the biscuit crumbs, cinnamon and margarine thoroughly and press into a 23 cm (9 inch) springform pan and bake crust for 8–10 minutes or until set. Cool.

3 Pour the orange juice into a small saucepan. Sprinkle the gelatine on top and let soften for 3 minutes.

4 Heat, stirring constantly, until the gelatine dissolves (about 6 minutes).

5 Blend the cheeses in a large bowl until smooth. Stir in the sweetener.

6 Add the gelatine mixture and blend until smooth.

7 Chill in the refrigerator for about 15 minutes.

8 Prepare the whipped topping mix according to the package directions, substituting the skimmed milk for water.

9 Fold the whipped topping into the cheese mixture. Stir in the chopped oranges.

10 Spoon into the prepared crust and spread evenly. Chill for 6 hours or overnight.

11 Decorate with orange sections and mint leaves.

Fresh Fruit Soufflé

per portion: 52 kcals • 4 g protein
• 0 g fat • 10 g CHO

Serves 6

450–900 g (1–2 lb) fruit (peaches, pears, blueberries, strawberries, raspberries)

artificial sweetener, to taste

cornflour

6 egg whites

caster or icing sugar

1 Cook fruit to make strong purée. Add a little artificial sweetener if necessary.

2 Thicken the fruit purée with cornflour, until it is the consistency of jam.

3 Whisk the egg whites until they form stiff peaks.

4 Gently fold the egg whites into the fruit purée.

5 Pour the mixture into a non-stick soufflé bowl dusted with caster or icing sugar.

6 Bake in a preheated oven at 180°C (350°F), Gas Mark 4, for 40–50 minutes, or until well risen (approximately double the size) and brown on top.

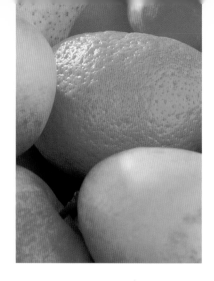

Sponge Cake Extraordinaire

per portion: 64 kcals • 2 g protein • 2 g fat • 11 g CHO

Serves 16

120 g (4 oz) sifted sugar

1 tsp lemon or orange rind, grated

3 egg yolks

4 tbs boiling water (or coffee)

1 tbs lemon juice (or 1 tsp vanilla essence or 3 drops anise oil)

85 g (3 oz) flour

1½ tsp baking powder

⅛ tsp salt

6 egg whites

1 Preheat the oven to 180°C (350°F), Gas Mark 4.

2 Sift sugar and stir in grated lemon or orange rind.

3 Beat the egg yolks until light. Beat in sugar gradually.

4 Beat the water (or coffee) into the yolks and sugar. Cool.

5 Stir in the lemon juice (or vanilla essence or anise).

6 Resift the flour with the baking powder and salt, and add gradually to the yolk mixture. Stir until perfectly blended.

7 Whip the egg whites just until stiff. Fold into the batter.

8 Bake in a 23 cm (9 inch) non-stick sandwich tin in a preheated oven for about 45 minutes.

9 Serve with berries or peaches, either fresh or stewed with no added sugar, with 2 tablespoons of virtually fat-free yogurt.

10 Alternatively, fill the centre with a variety of cut fresh fruit just before serving. For very special occasions, ice with Vanilla Foam Icing (page 61), with or without the filling of fresh fruit.

Vanilla Foam Icing

per portion: 75 kcals • 0.5 g protein • 0 g fat • 25 g CHO

Serves 16

2 egg whites

340 g (12 oz) sugar

5 tbs cold water

¼ tsp cream of tartar

1 tsp vanilla essence

1 Place the egg whites, sugar, water and cream of tartar in the top section of a double boiler. Beat until thoroughly blended.

2 Place over rapidly boiling water and beat constantly with a rotary beater for 7 minutes.

3 Remove from the heat. Add the vanilla essence.

4 Continue beating until the icing is a thick consistency for spreading.

5 Ice the cake only after it is cool. Icing the Sponge Cake Extraordinaire (page 60) makes a very elegant dessert.

Lemon Foam Icing

per portion: 100 kcals • 0.5 g protein • 0 g fat • 25 g CHO

Serves 16

Make as Vanilla Foam Icing, but replace 5 tablespoons cold water with 3 tablespoons cold water, 2 tablespoons lemon juice and ¼ teaspoon grated lemon rind.

Orange Foam Icing

per portion: 84 kcals • 6 g protein 0 g fat • 27 g CHO

Serves 16

Make as Vanilla Foam Icing, but replace 5 tablespoons cold water with 4 tablespoons orange juice, 1 tablespoon lemon juice and ½ teaspoon grated orange rind.

Rainbow Ice

per portion: 71 kcals • 3 g protein • 0 g fat • 15 g CHO

Serves 6

½ tsp powdered gelatine

4 tbs cold water

2–3 tsp artificial sweetener (to taste) or 2 tbs honey

2 tbs lemon juice

6 tbs orange juice

225 ml (8 fl oz) fresh peach purée

225 ml (8 fl oz) fresh kiwi purée

225 ml (8 fl oz) fresh raspberry purée

1 Soak the gelatine in the cold water in a saucepan for 5 minutes. Heat to dissolve the gelatine.

2 Add sweetener to each of the fruit purées.

3 Mix the lemon and orange juices and add one-third to each sweetened purée.

4 Pour the peach purée into a glass loaf tin lined with waxed paper. Freeze until hard.

5 Put the kiwi purée on top of the frozen peach purée and freeze until hard.

6 Finally, layer the raspberry purée on top. Freeze until hard.

Warm Apple Delight

per portion: 56 kcals • 1 g protein • 0 g fat • 14 g CHO

Serves 2

2 red apples, cored and cut in half (with skin)

1 can diet black cherry or strawberry cola

pinch of artificial sweetener

pinch of cinnamon

1 Place the apple in a baking dish skin-side down. Pour the cola over apple.

2 Sprinkle with sweetener and cinnamon.

3 Bake in a preheated oven at 180°C (350°F), Gas Mark 4, for 25–30 minutes.

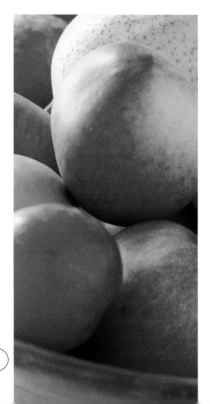

Oranges Floridean

per portion: 119 kcals • 2 g protein • 0 g fat • 21 g CHO

Serves 8

8 navel oranges

285 g (10 oz) frozen raspberries

340 g (12 oz) fresh raspberries

120 ml (4 fl oz) Drambuie or grenadine

1 tsp arrowroot

mint leaves, to decorate

1 Peel the oranges, removing the white pith and the skin, and slice them horizontally. Put them aside in a large, flat bowl.

2 In a blender, purée the frozen raspberries and half of the fresh raspberries.

3 Strain to remove all seeds.

4 Add the Drambuie or grenadine and heat for 3 minutes in a saucepan. Add the arrowroot and stir to thicken. Let cool.

5 Place 4 orange slices in individual dessert plates and top with 2 tablespoons of purée. Decorate with mint leaves and the remaining fresh raspberries.

6 Chill for at least 4 hours before serving.

Whipped Fruit Wonder

per portion: 171 kcals • 12 g protein • 7 g fat • 16 g CHO

Serves 2

1 tsp powdered gelatine

75–120 ml (3–4 fl oz) fruit juice

4 fresh apricots or 2 fresh peaches, peeled and puréed with 1 tsp lemon juice or 1 small jar prepared baby food (apricots, prunes, apple sauce, peaches, etc.)

1 tsp artificial sweetener

½ tsp vanilla essence

120 g (4 oz) low-fat ricotta cheese

120 g (4 oz) low-fat yogurt

1 Soak the gelatine in the fruit juice. Heat over hot water to dissolve.

2 Add the puréed fruit, half of the sweetener and vanilla. Chill until the mixture becomes syrupy in consistency.

3 Whip in a chilled bowl until the gelatine has doubled in bulk. Pour into individual dessert dishes and chill for at least 4 hours.

4 In a bowl, mix the ricotta cheese and the yogurt with the remaining sweetener, to use as a topping. Decorate with slices of fruit.

The Life of the Party

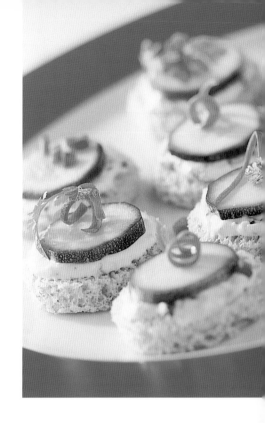

Even special occasions can be celebrated with fewer kilocalories! Since preparing for parties is always last minute and hectic, it is best to prepare as much as possible in advance. You can also serve finger-sized Special Sandwiches (page 35).

Courgette Gondolier

per portion: 21 kcals • 1 g protein • 1 g fat • 3 g CHO

Makes 36

1 medium courgette, sliced

120 ml (4 fl oz) vinegar

120 ml (4 fl oz) water

6 ice cubes

60 g (2 oz) semi-skimmed ricotta cheese

2 tbs Mayo-n-eze (page 46)

1 tsp finely chopped onion

½ tsp finely chopped fresh watercress

⅛ tsp dried chervil

⅛ tsp dried savory

1 tsp lemon juice

dash of hot sauce

9 slices thinly sliced wholemeal bread

pimento slices, to garnish

1 Combine the courgette, vinegar, water and ice cubes in a bowl. Let stand for 30 minutes.

2 Mix together the ricotta cheese, Mayo-n-eze, onion, watercress, chervil, savory, lemon juice and hot sauce. Cover and chill.

3 Remove the crust from the bread. Cut four 3.5 cm (1½ inch) rounds from each bread slice. Spread ½ teaspoon ricotta mixture on each round. Top with a slice of courgette. Garnish with pimento slices.

Peking Purée

per portion: 15 kcals • 0 g protein • 1 g fat • 0 g CHO

Serves 50

120 ml (4 fl oz) plain low-fat yogurt

120 ml (4 fl oz) Mayo-n-eze (page 46)

1 tbs sesame seeds, toasted

2 tbs reduced-sodium soy sauce

2 tbs Worcestershire sauce

1½ tsp ground ginger

1 Thoroughly mix all the ingredients in a small bowl.

2 Cover and refrigerate for at least 4 hours before serving.

Fruit Kebabs

per portion: 44 kcals • 1 g protein • 0 g fat • 10 g CHO

Serves 16

2 apples, peeled and cut into 2 cm (¾ inch) cubes

225 g (8 oz) pineapple cubes (fresh or canned)

140 g (5 oz) fresh strawberries, stems removed and cut in half

170 g (6 oz) cantaloupe melon balls or cubes

170 g (6 oz) honeydew melon balls or cubes

170 g (6 oz) watermelon balls or cubes (in season)

1 fresh pineapple to serve

1 Dip each apple cube into lemon juice to prevent discoloration.

2 Put 1 piece of fruit on to each wooden skewer, alternating colours, ending with a strawberry at the tip.

3 Serve round a whole pineapple, with some skewers decoratively stuck into the pineapple.

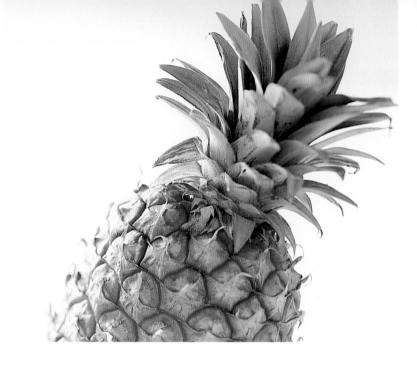

Courgette Zaragone

per portion, including toast: 24 kcals • 1 g protein • 1 g fat • 4 g CHO

Serves 8

2 courgettes

½ tsp dried oregano

1 tbs chopped spring onion

½ tsp salt

¼ tsp black pepper

¼ tsp olive oil

1 tsp vinegar

2 tsp chopped coriander leaves

parsley, to garnish

1 Wash the courgettes (with the skin) and grate.

2 Add all the other ingredients and mix well.

3 Serve on quartered, thin slices of toasted wholegrain bread. Garnish with parsley.

Yellow Fin Mousse

per tablespoon: 8 kcals • 1 g protein • 0 g fat • 1 g CHO

Makes 22 tablespoons

100 g (3½ oz) water-packed canned tuna, drained and flaked

85 ml (3 fl oz) low-fat plain yogurt

15 g (½ oz) celery, finely chopped

1 apple, pared and finely chopped

1 large pickle, finely chopped

1 tsp lemon juice

pinch of paprika

pinch of black pepper

1 Mash the tuna in a bowl with a fork until smooth.

2 Stir in first the yogurt, then the remaining ingredients.

3 Serve on biscuits garnished with parsley and a wedge of cherry tomato, or as a dip with crudités. This is also excellent to serve with lettuce as a tuna salad.

Chicken Bites Orientale

per portion: 19 kcals • 4 g protein • 0.5 g fat • 0 g CHO

Serves 50

4 chicken breast halves (about 750 g (1 lb 10 oz)

400 ml (14 fl oz) water

2 tbs reduced-sodium soy sauce

1 tbs Worcestershire sauce

225 g (8 oz) large fresh spinach leaves, trimmed and washed

cos lettuce

Peking Purée (page 63)

1 Skin chicken and trim excess fat.

2 Combine water, soy sauce and Worcestershire sauce in a large frying pan and bring to a boil. Add the chicken; cover and simmer over low heat for 20 minutes or until chicken is tender.

3 Remove the bones and cut the meat into 2.5 cm (1 inch) cubes.

4 Place the spinach leaves on a covered steaming rack over boiling water. Cover and steam for 1 minute.

5 Place 1 cube of chicken on each spinach leaf. Roll once, fold the leaf in on both sides, and continue rolling around the chicken cube. Secure the spinach leaf with a cocktail stick.

6 Cover and chill thoroughly. Serve on lettuce with Peking Purée.

Crunchy Crudités

per portion: 21 kcals • 1 g protein • 0 g fat • 4 g CHO

For an especially elegant presentation, cut with a special ridged blade:

carrots, celery, courgettes

slices of green, yellow, and red pepper

cauliflower and broccoli florets

mangetout (snow pea pods)

cherry tomatoes

mushrooms

Arrange decoratively around a dish of dip, salad dressing, unsweetened apple sauce minimally seasoned with cinnamon, or non-oil salsa.

Velouté of Onion

per tablespoon: • 19 kcals • 2 g protein • 0 g fat • 3 g CHO

Makes 20 tablespoons

1 packet dried onion soup

450 ml (¾ pint) very low-fat yogurt

Mix the dried onion soup with the yogurt. Chill for 2 hours before serving.

Tomatoes Napolitano

per portion, including toast: 21 kcals • 1 g protein • 1 g fat • 3 g CHO

Serves 8

2 tomatoes

½ teaspoon dried oregano

1 tbs chopped spring onion

¼ tsp black pepper

¼ tsp olive oil

1 tsp vinegar

parsley, to garnish

1 Dip the tomatoes into hot water and remove the skin. Dice.

2 Combine with all the other ingredients and mix well.

3 Serve on thin quarters of toasted wholegrain bread. Garnish with parsley.

Fresh Ricotta

per tablespoon: • 10 kcals • 1 g protein • 1 g fat • 1 g CHO

Makes 16 tablespoons

175 g (6 oz) low-fat ricotta cheese

40 g (1½ oz) sweet mustard pickles

Mix the ricotta cheese with the mustard pickles. Chill for 2 hours before serving.

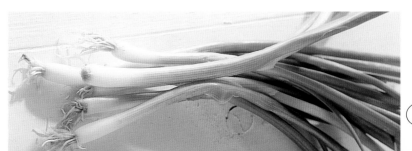

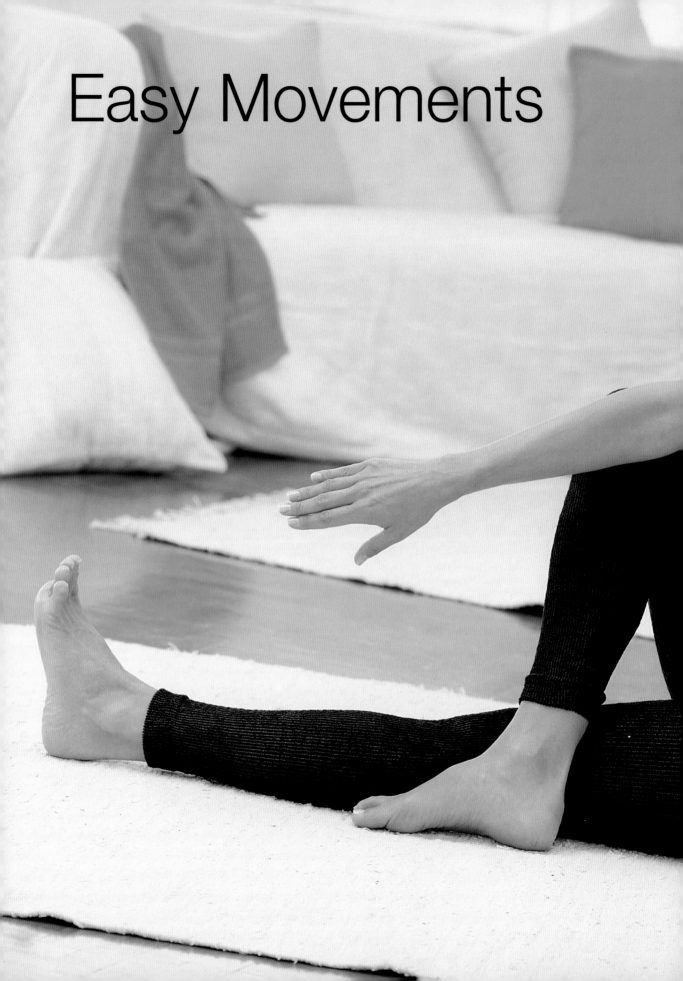

Easy Movements

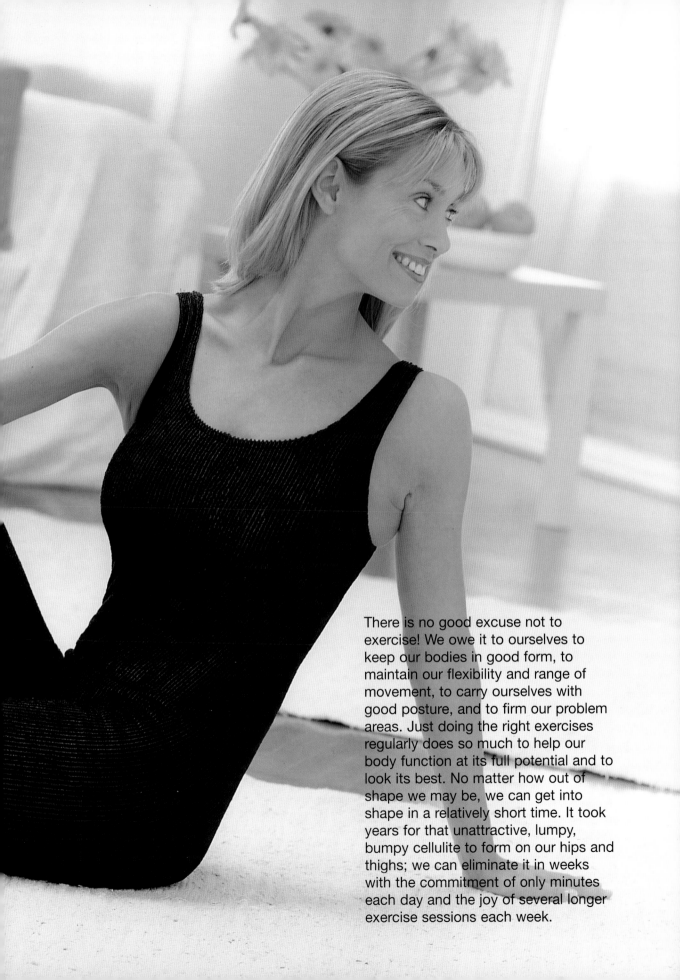

There is no good excuse not to exercise! We owe it to ourselves to keep our bodies in good form, to maintain our flexibility and range of movement, to carry ourselves with good posture, and to firm our problem areas. Just doing the right exercises regularly does so much to help our body function at its full potential and to look its best. No matter how out of shape we may be, we can get into shape in a relatively short time. It took years for that unattractive, lumpy, bumpy cellulite to form on our hips and thighs; we can eliminate it in weeks with the commitment of only minutes each day and the joy of several longer exercise sessions each week.

The Exercises

You will see a change in your body by following this easy, four-part routine:

1 The **Pressometric** isometric movements, which can be done anywhere, anytime, give your thighs, buttocks and arms a svelte line.

2 The **Twelve-Minute Miracle** daily exercise routine is designed to resculpt cellulite-laden areas. These subtle, controlled, non-strenuous movements preceded by the **Streamline Stretches** are based on yoga and ballet.

3 The **Thigh Thinners** provide a special toning workout that takes about 20 minutes by expanding on the **Twelve-Minute Miracle**. To achieve the best results, follow this routine at least two or three times each week. Also based on yoga and ballet, these exercises give the quickest and most effective results in refining your silhouette and adding elegance to your everyday posture and movement.

4 Many different **Aerobic Exercises** are described, so that you can design an activity that you can integrate into your schedule two or three times each week. You will learn not only to walk for your errands, but to "power walk". You will also find time to enjoy dancing, jumping, skipping, bicycling or swimming.

Each long journey begins with the first step

The toughest part of starting any exercise programme is motivating yourself to begin. We all have busy schedules, with little, if any, spare time. Joining a health club or an exercise class is not only inconvenient and expensive, but also intimidating, especially if you are self-conscious about your cellulite. I don't discourage you from joining a gym – I just want to give you a super-effective exercise routine that you can easily do in the privacy of your own home. It's best to keep to a schedule; exercise at a specific time, convenient to you. I do my short daily routine just after rising in the morning. If you start work

very early or take children to school, perhaps you should exercise at noon, later in the afternoon, or just before bed.

Contrary to some opinion, exercising just before sleeping is beneficial, especially doing the stretching routines that follow. These exercises increase your metabolism (with additional benefit, even as you sleep), and as they help you relax, you sleep better. And you can always find time late at night for a short routine!

To see a change in your body soon, do:

Each day:
> **Pressometrics**
> **Streamline Stretches**
> **Twelve-Minute Miracle**

Monday, Wednesday, Friday:
> **Thigh Thinners**

Tuesday or Thursday, Saturday, Sunday:
> **Aerobics**

To give health and vitality, exercise must become a permanent part of your life. Movement preserves youth; if you do not move and stretch enough, your body ages prematurely. By tailoring your own programme, you will make your exercise routine an enjoyable and convenient treat! Don't put it off for another day!

Positive Posture

Have you ever glimpsed your reflection in a window and realized that you were slumping? Fortunately, if you do the exercises you are about to learn, that will not happen! This routine tones your muscles and keeps you elegantly erect without conscious effort. Do an experiment right now. Stand in front of the mirror in a bathing suit or leotard, facing sideways. Contract your buttocks and tuck in your stomach in the **Hip Hugger** (see page 71). You will immediately appear thinner. This contracted position also corrects any exaggerated inward curvature of the lower back. This is important, especially if you wear high heels which can cause an unattractive protrusion of the stomach and buttocks. Consciously pulling in your stomach is the single best exercise to flatten your abdomen. This isometric contraction, which you can do anywhere and at any time, beats hundreds of daily sit-ups!

Now use a second mirror to look at your rear view. As you tighten your buttocks in the **Hip Hugger**, you see that the sides of your thighs have a smoother line, your buttocks move up, and you look like the "after" of surgical liposuction – all from just standing straight with an isometric pelvic contraction.

The Puppet Posture Rule

The secret of good posture is to sit, stand and walk tall. To achieve this without strain, pretend you are suspended like a puppet by a string from the top of your head. This image automatically causes you to straighten your neck, shoulders and back without artificial contortion. Your shoulders are relaxed and your chest is naturally lifted. When you sit, you will not slump habitually to one side (which can stretch the muscles on one side and contract those on the other to create scoliosis, or curvature of the spine). Instead, your weight will be equally distributed on your pelvic bone.

Remember, most of us sit for up to eight or even 14 hours each day – in the office, in the car or train, at meals, in front of the TV. Your posture is important – to improve breathing, to increase energy, and to look much better.

Look at the photographs on the right, to see how much better you appear, with back and shoulders straight, when you follow the **Puppet Posture Rule**. In addition, when you stand and walk "tight", with the **Hip Hugger** in mind, your abdomen is flat, your buttocks are higher, and your thighs appear thinner.

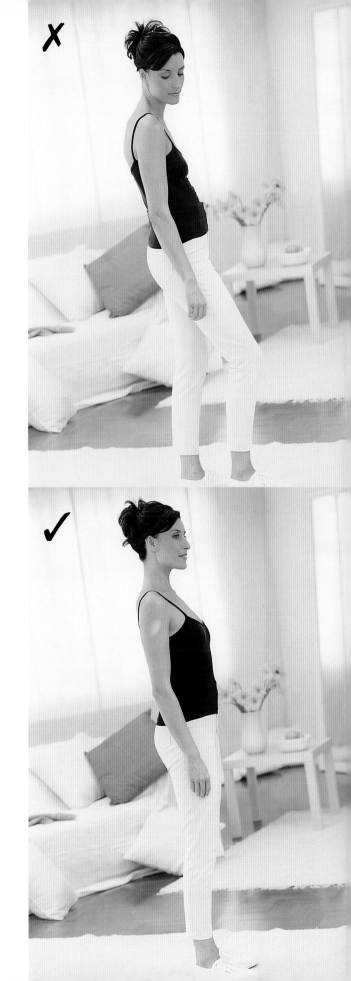

Pressometrics

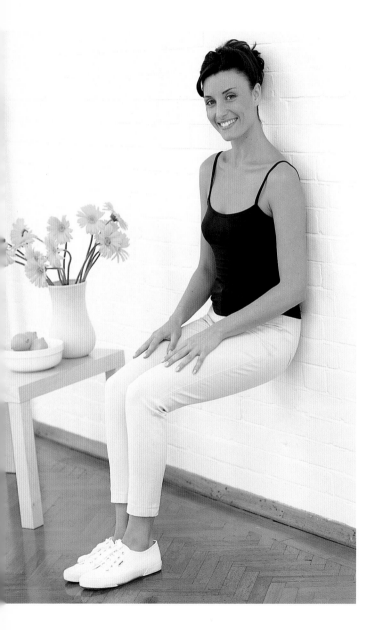

You can truly achieve a slimmer line to your thighs and buttocks within weeks without taking time from your routine activities or buying expensive equipment. These exercises are carefully controlled, subtle movements that are not difficult, and they are fun! The special advantage of these **Pressometrics** is that you can integrate them into your daily activities. They do not tire you; in fact, you can use them at any time during the day if you feel fatigued or bored to give you energy. As you brush your teeth, shower, dry your hair, cook, wait for a lift, bus or train, talk on the telephone, work at your desk, or watch television, you can reshape your body. Even during tiring meetings or in a traffic jam, there is a toning **Pressometric** you can do. You can become happy and energized by challenging yourself to do each movement for a longer count than you achieved on the previous occasion. These movements will become second nature to you, a permanent part of you life – and so will your new svelte silhouette!

Pressometric Tips

1 Initially hold each contraction for a count of 10. Gradually work your way up to a count of 30.

2 Start with three repetitions of each contraction. Increase gradually to 10 repetitions at a time.

3 Increase the number of sets you do each day, especially those that act on your particular trouble spots.

4 Think about the muscles as you contract.

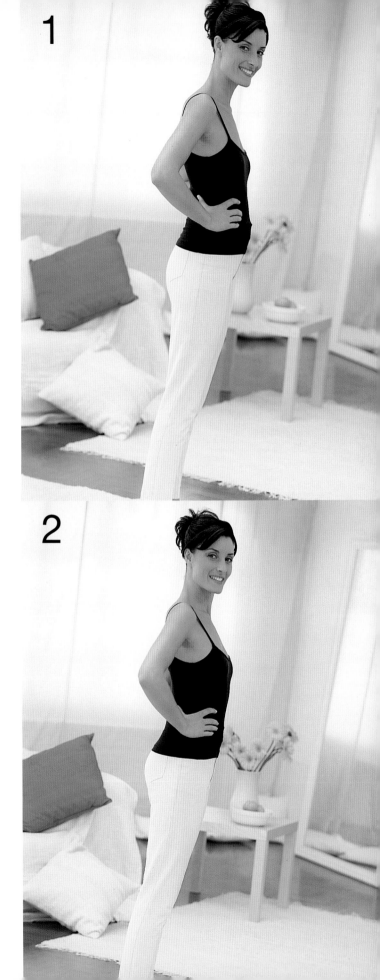

Hip Hugger

The **Hip Hugger**, also known as the **Pelvic Tuck**, is the easiest and most effective exercise for toning your thighs and buttocks. It is possibly the single most effective "cellulite burner".

1 Stand with your feet shoulder width apart and your hands on your waist.

2 Contract your abdominal muscles, and squeeze your buttocks together (hard!). Your pelvis will move forward so that you look thinner and more toned instantly. You will also feel the squeeze in your outer and inner thighs.

3 Pretend you are grasping a pencil between your buttocks, or a thin piece of paper between your thighs.

4 Hold this contraction initially for a count of 10 and work your way up to a count of 30.

The Achilles Step-Up

This stretch is especially important for us women who often wear chic high heels, resulting in contraction of the Achilles tendon. This simple exercise can be done on any stair or even on a large book. By just repeating five times in several pauses during your day, you will see the silhouette of your thighs and buttocks become sleeker.

1 Place the balls of your feet on the edge of a stair or book, with your heels hanging down over the edge. Stand straight with your buttocks squeezed together and your abdomen pulled into the **Hip Hugger**. If you have difficulty balancing, hold on to a railing or a bureau. Stretch for at least 20 seconds.

2 Stretch for at least 20 seconds. Concentrate on the pull in the back of your calf and thigh and on the contraction of your buttocks and abdomen. Lower your right heel below the level of your toes and raise your left heel.

3 Now lower your right heel below the level of your toes and raise your left heel.

4 If you can keep your balance by holding a support, repeat with both feet simultaneously.

Repeat: start with three repetitions of stepping left, then right, then three repetitions lowering both heels. Increase to 10 repetitions left and right, 10 repetitions both feet.

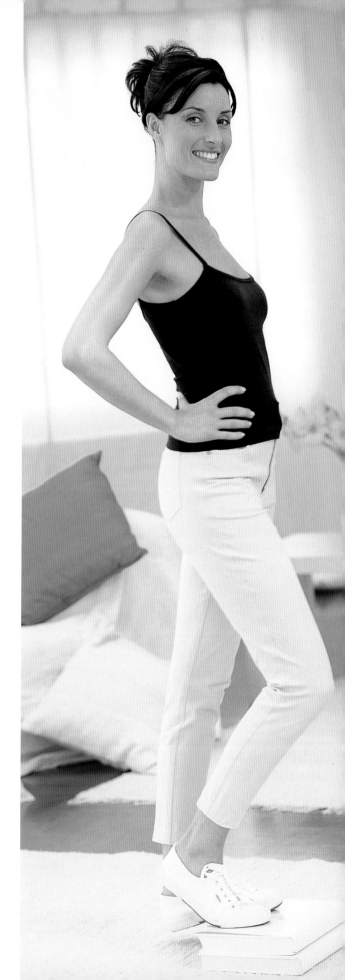

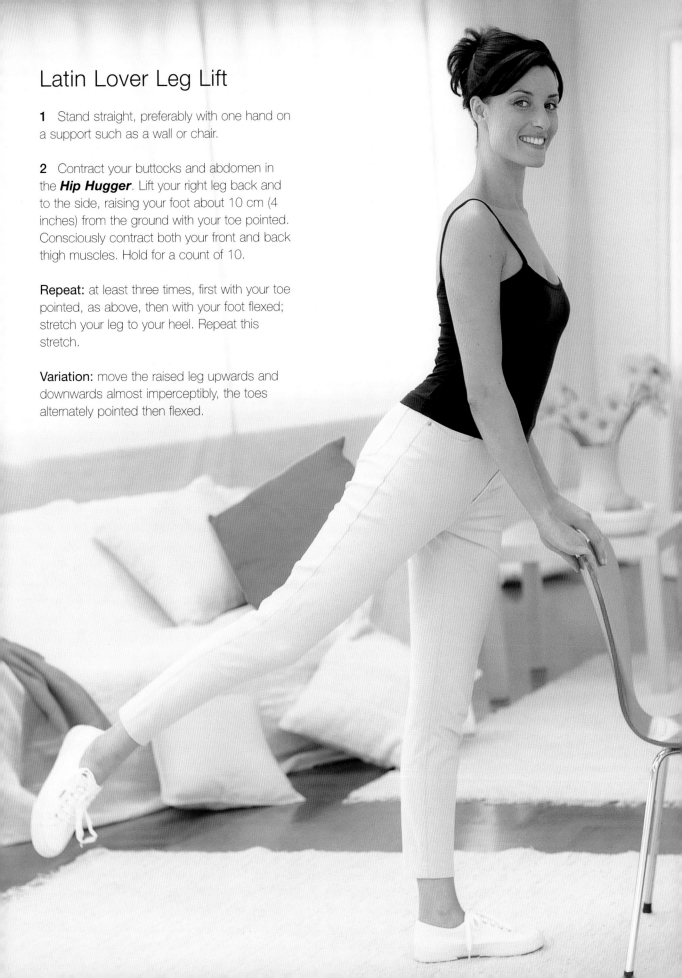

Latin Lover Leg Lift

1   Stand straight, preferably with one hand on a support such as a wall or chair.

2   Contract your buttocks and abdomen in the **_Hip Hugger_**. Lift your right leg back and to the side, raising your foot about 10 cm (4 inches) from the ground with your toe pointed. Consciously contract both your front and back thigh muscles. Hold for a count of 10.

Repeat: at least three times, first with your toe pointed, as above, then with your foot flexed; stretch your leg to your heel. Repeat this stretch.

Variation: move the raised leg upwards and downwards almost imperceptibly, the toes alternately pointed then flexed.

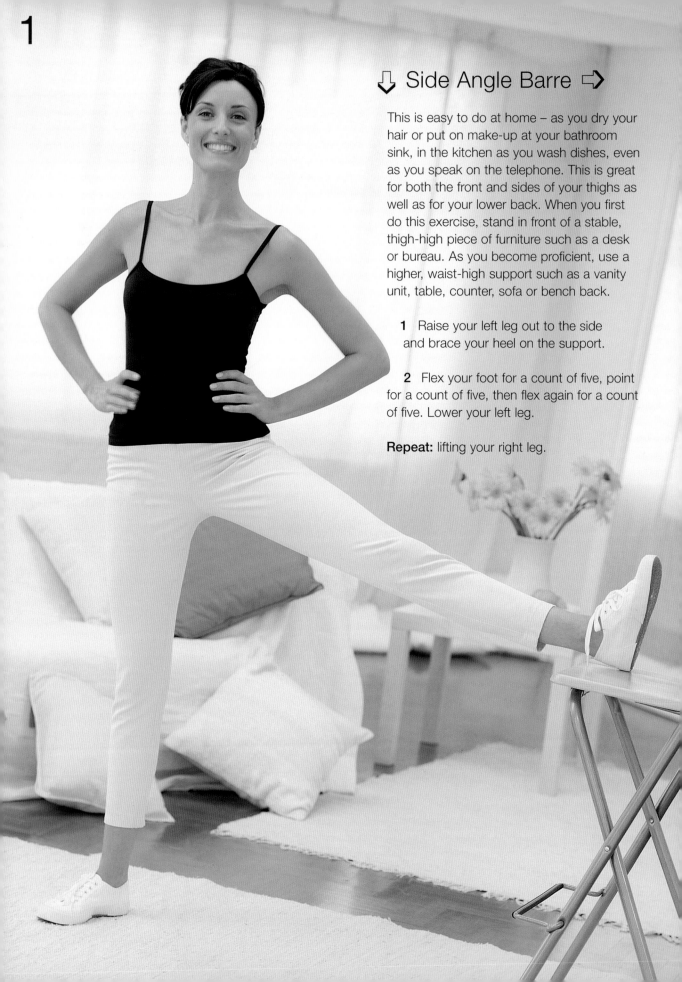

⬇ Side Angle Barre ⇨

This is easy to do at home – as you dry your hair or put on make-up at your bathroom sink, in the kitchen as you wash dishes, even as you speak on the telephone. This is great for both the front and sides of your thighs as well as for your lower back. When you first do this exercise, stand in front of a stable, thigh-high piece of furniture such as a desk or bureau. As you become proficient, use a higher, waist-high support such as a vanity unit, table, counter, sofa or bench back.

1 Raise your left leg out to the side and brace your heel on the support.

2 Flex your foot for a count of five, point for a count of five, then flex again for a count of five. Lower your left leg.

Repeat: lifting your right leg.

2

⬇ Front Angle Barre

1 Stand leg length away from a stable
support as before. Raise your left leg to the
front and brace your heel on the support. Lean
over and grasp your heel with both hands to
increase the stretch.

2 Lean over and try to touch your forehead to
your knee cap. Flex your foot for a count of
five, point for a count of five, then flex for a
count of five. Lower your left leg.

Repeat: lifting your right leg.

1

2

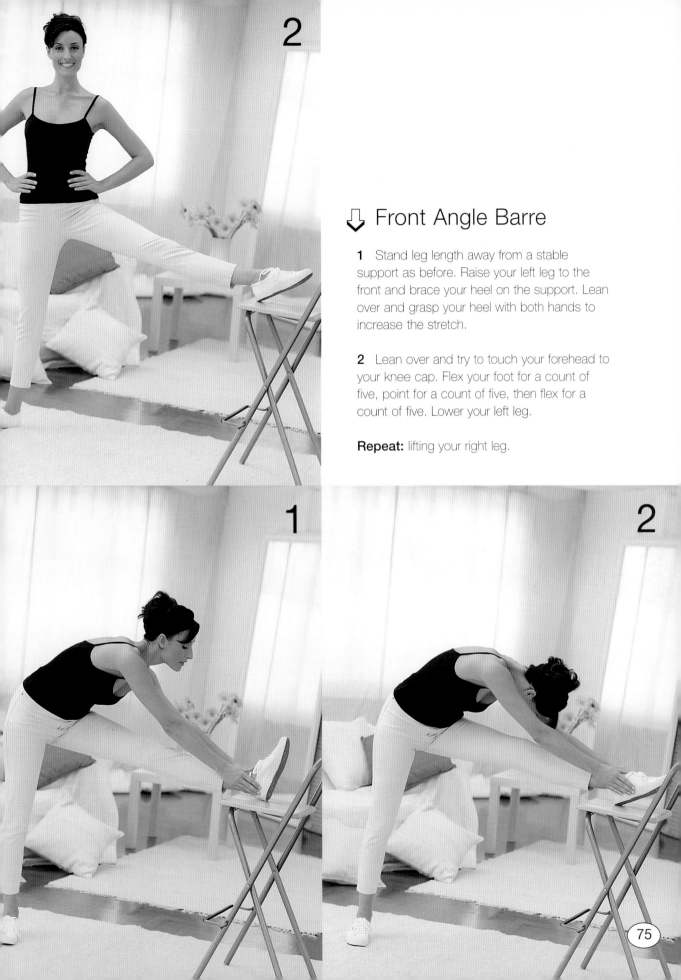

The Invisible Chair

This exercise makes telephone time become a super toning session – you must simply sit on an invisible chair!

1   Lean your back against a wall, flattening your spine against the wall as you pull your stomach into the *Hip Hugger* and squeeze your buttocks together.

2   Keeping your knees together, lower your body down the wall until your knees are bent at a 135°–90° angle. (As you improve you will sit lower with your knees at the 90° angle as shown.) You are now sitting on an invisible chair!

3   Hold for at least 20 seconds; work up to one full minute.

Repeat: three times; increase to five times.

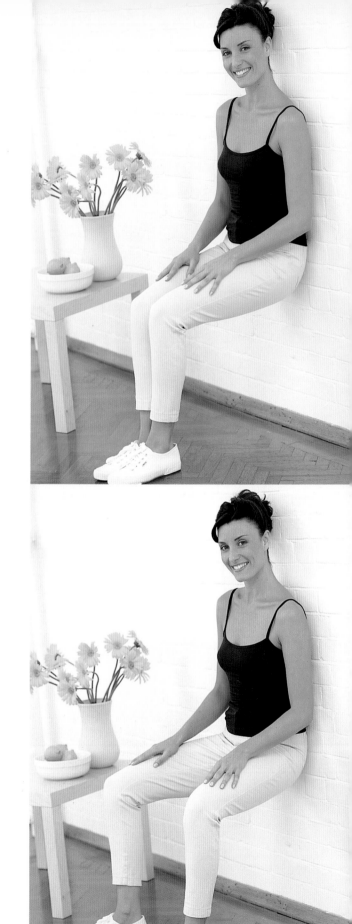

The Invisible Bench

1   Lean your back against a wall with your feet shoulder width apart. (As you improve, you can spread your knees up to 15 cm (6 inches) wider apart than your shoulders. Flatten your spine against the wall as you pull your stomach into the *Hip Hugger* and squeeze your buttocks together.

2   Lower your body along the wall until your knees are bent to a 135°–90° angle. You are now sitting on an invisible bench! As you improve you will sit lower with your knees at a 90° angle as shown.

3   Hold for at least 20 seconds; work up to one full minute.

Repeat: three times; increase to five times.

Ball Crusher

This is the best single exercise that you can do for your inner thighs. Because it is squeezable, a child's ball is great to use for this exercise, preferably about 10–15 cm (4–6 inches) in diameter. Just keep your ball near the places you habitually sit.

1 Sit up straight at the edge of your chair. With your feet together, place the ball between your knees and keep it in place by applying pressure with your inner thighs.

2 Squeeze the ball as hard as you can, feeling the contraction of your inner thighs.

3 Hold for a count of 10, then relax, but keep the ball in place.

Repeat: at least three times.

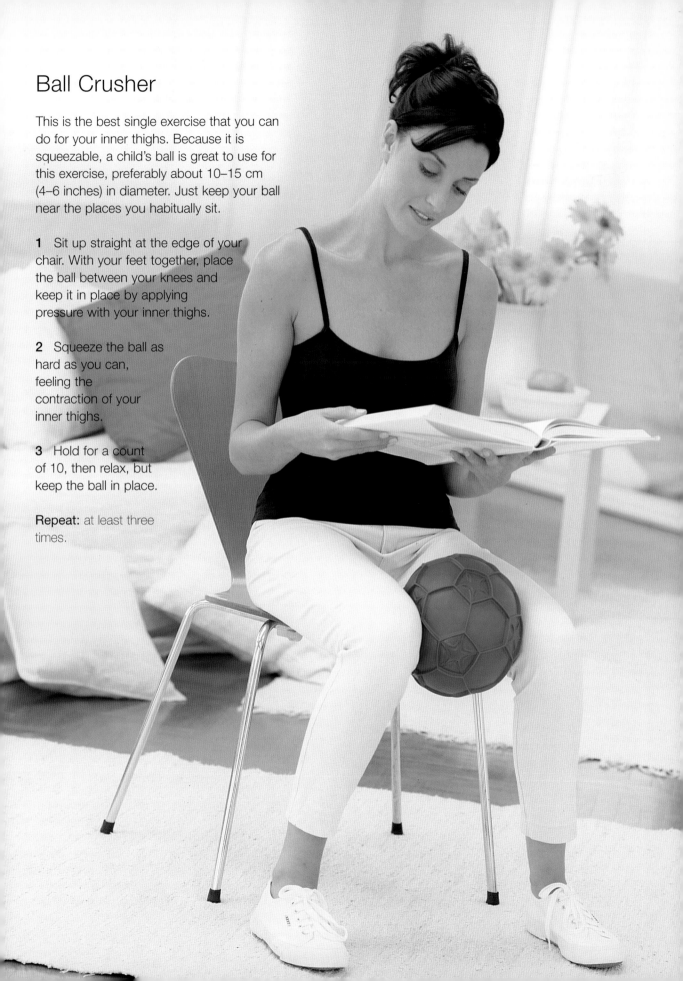

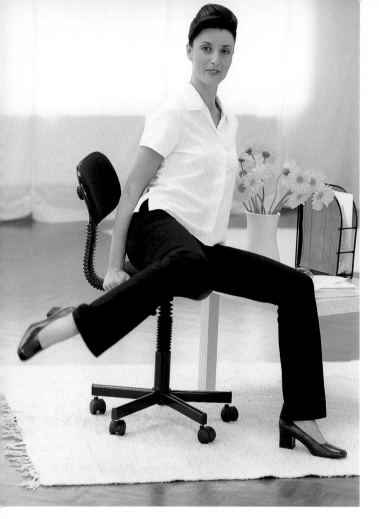

⇐ Saddle Battle

1 Sit forward on a chair without arms, close to the right corner. With straight arms, grasp the bottom or back of the chair on each side.

2 Place your left foot flat in front of the chair, slightly towards the right side. Lift your right leg back along the right side of the chair with your knee bent, so your lower leg is nearly parallel to the side of the chair.

3 Keeping your back straight, tuck your pelvis forward and think of pointing your knee into the floor while raising your foot to the ceiling.

4 Move your right knee gently back about 7.5 cm (3 inches). Hold for a count of 10, then return to the initial position. The movement is quite small; it should be done smoothly.

Repeat: three times; sit close to the left front corner of the chair and repeat for the left leg.

⇒ Suspended Animation

Joan Crawford is said to have been able to sit through an entire meal doing this exercise!

1 Sit forward in your chair so that you do not touch the back. Keep your legs together with your knees bent and your feet flat on the floor.

2 Now raise your feet about 7.5 cm (3 inches) off the floor. Keep your back straight and try to relax your arms so that the muscular contraction is entirely in your buttocks and thighs. This also strengthens your abdominal muscles to give you a flatter stomach.

3 Hold for a count of at least five; then try to work up to a count of 10.

Repeat: three times.

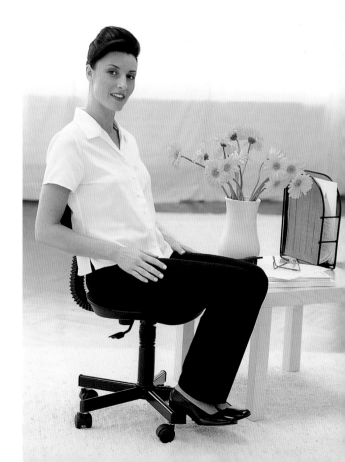

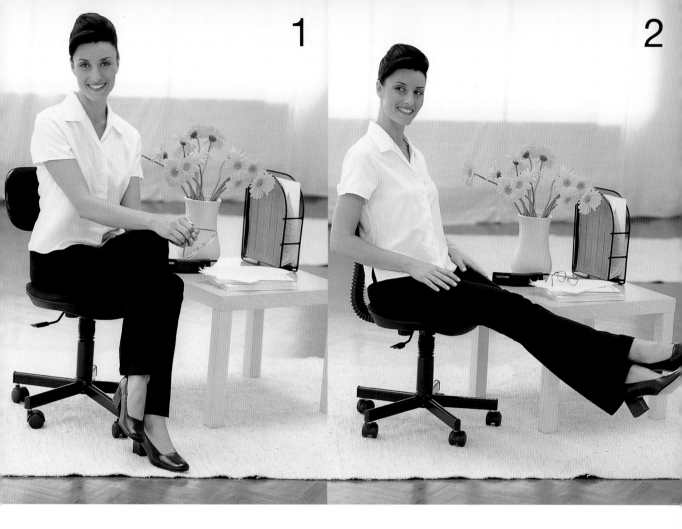

⇧ Suspended Relaxation

This is a variant of **Suspended Animation**, which Joan Crawford used to such good effect to make a meeting or a social meal into an exercise.

1   Sit comfortably in a chair. Cross your ankles and knees, pressing your left ankle and left knee over the right. Squeeze your lower legs together. Feel the contraction of your thigh muscles! Hold for a count of 10.

2   With your legs still crossed, extend them straight out in front of you. Again squeeze your ankles and knees together for a count of 10.

Repeat: to the other side, crossing your right ankle in front of the left.

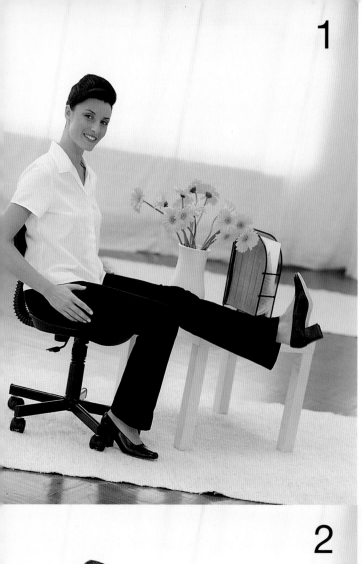

1

⬅ Suspended Flextension

1 Sit comfortably in a chair with your feet flat on the floor, with your abdomen pulled in and your buttocks squeezed together tightly. Keeping your left ankle flexed, raise your left leg, extending it straight in front of you. Squeeze your knees together, concentrating on your inner thighs. Hold with your left foot flexed for a count of five, then pointed for a count of five, then flexed for a count of five. Lower your left leg to the floor. Repeat with the right.

2 Extend both legs in front of you. Squeeze your knees together, concentrating on your inner thighs.

3 Hold with ankles flexed for a count of five, then pointed for five, then flexed for five.

4 Lower both legs to the floor.

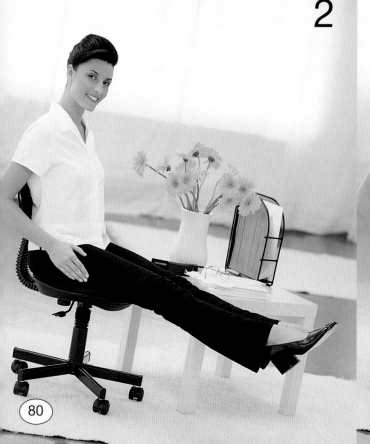

2

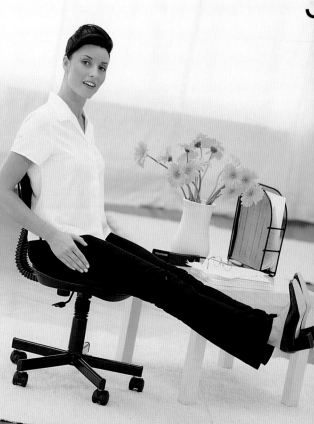

3

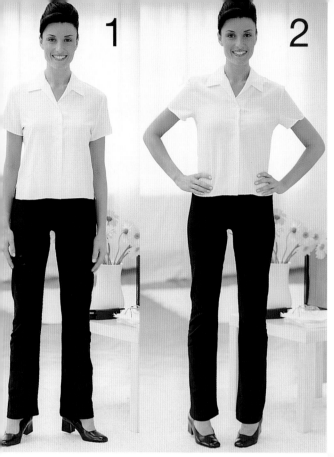

⬇ Knee Cap Kiss

This is an easy but effective exercise, perfect for when you are sitting in a compact space like a train or plane or when you are on the telephone. Make sure that the chair you sit on is not too high; you should be able to sit with your feet flat on the floor.

1   Sit up straight with your knees together and your feet slightly apart. Squeeze your knees together, feeling the contraction of your inner thighs. Simultaneously contract the muscles of your abdomen and buttocks as in the **Hip Hugger** (see page 71).

2   Hold for a count of 10, then relax.

Repeat: at least three times.

⬆ Elevator Wait Lift

1   Stand with your pelvis contracted in the **Hip Hugger** position (see page 71), with your heels about 15 cm (6 inches) apart and your toes facing diagonally out. Raise your heels, supporting yourself by lightly holding on to the wall if necessary. Concentrate on the muscle tension in the front and the sides of your thighs. Hold for a count of 10, then return to the starting position.

2   Stand with toes together and heels pointing out. Raise your heels for a count of 10. Concentrate on the muscle tension in the back of your thighs.

3   Stand with your feet straight forward. Raise your heels for a count of 10, concentrating on the muscle contraction in the sides and back of your thighs.

Repeat: three times with toes facing out, three times with toes facing in, three times with toes facing forward.

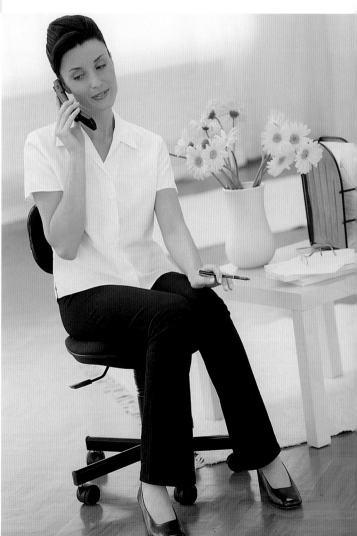

⬇ Torso Twister

This enhances your posture and slims your upper arms and those unsightly love handles on your back as it contours your thighs.

1 Sit up straight in a chair, crossing your left leg over your right knee.

2 Straighten your left arm and press the back of your left hand against your left knee (palm in).

3 Turn to the right as far as you can from your waist up, putting your right forearm along the back of the chair. Turn your head to look as far over your right shoulder as possible, maximizing the stretch. Concentrate on pushing your thighs to the right as you press the back of your hand to the left. Hold for a count of 20.

Repeat: on the other side.

⬇ Flapper

1 Intertwine your fingers behind your head, elbows bent to the side.

2 Push your upper arms back gently as if trying to make your shoulder blades touch. Hold for a count of 10.

Repeat: three times.

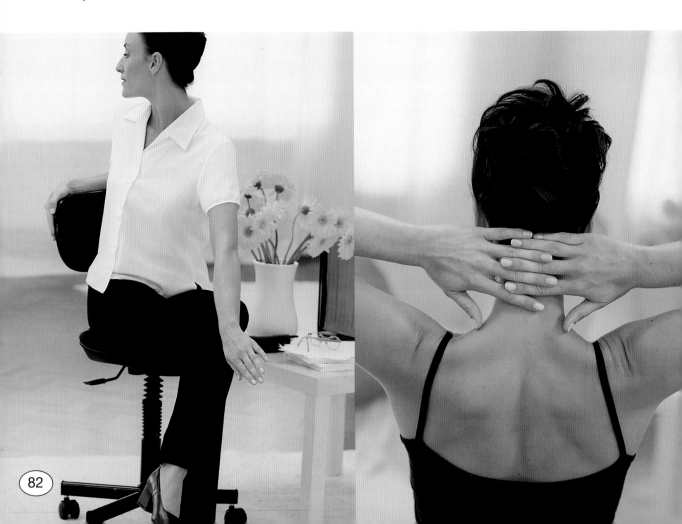

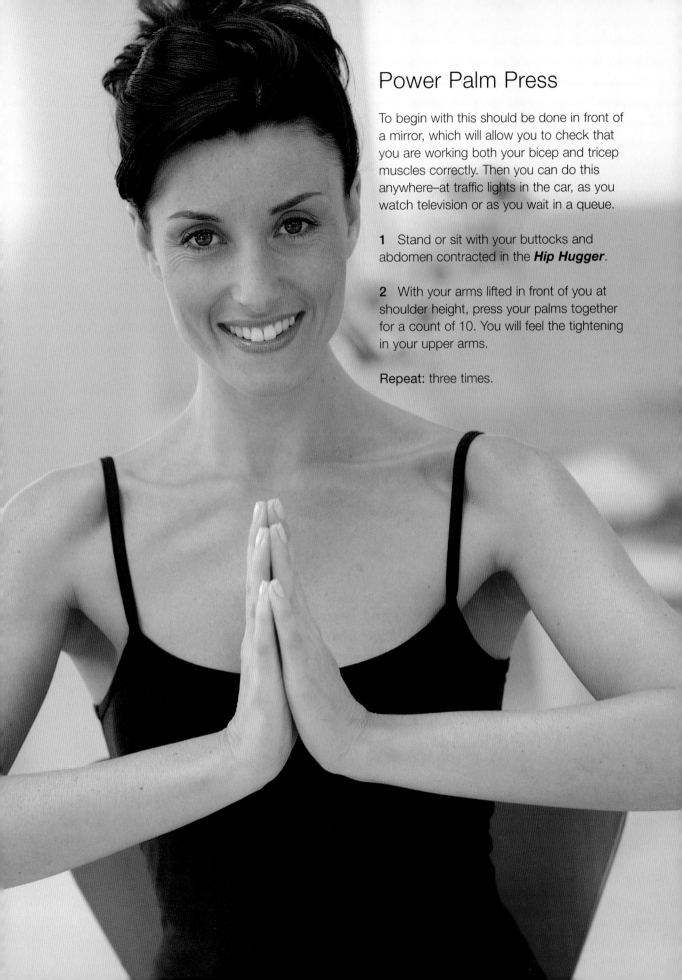

Power Palm Press

To begin with this should be done in front of a mirror, which will allow you to check that you are working both your bicep and tricep muscles correctly. Then you can do this anywhere–at traffic lights in the car, as you watch television or as you wait in a queue.

1   Stand or sit with your buttocks and abdomen contracted in the *Hip Hugger*.

2   With your arms lifted in front of you at shoulder height, press your palms together for a count of 10. You will feel the tightening in your upper arms.

Repeat: three times.

Streamline Stretches

Think of how a cat awakens with a long stretch. Stretching eases the transition from rest to motion. Stretching is also the best method to resculpt your body to eliminate the appearance of cellulite. Elongating the muscles and the overlying layer of fat decreases the uneven surface appearance of cellulite. In contrast, building muscles worsens the appearance of cellulite in two ways: by adding bulk and by pushing on overlying cellulite to accentuate the dimply surface.

The **Streamline Stretches** you are about to learn not only help your joints prepare for more strenuous exercise, but also directly improve your posture and give you a thinner, smoother contour. In performing these **Streamline Stretches**, move slowly into the stretch position and hold initially for a count of ten, increasing this count each day if there is no strain. This is called "static stretching". Ideally one can improve flexibility by extending the muscles as far as comfortably possible with each stretch. But remember that in stretching it is not true that "the more it hurts, the better it is." When done correctly, stretches feel really good!

An alternative to holding the stretch is to pulsate gently. However, do avoid bouncing in and out of the stretched position using unrestrained momentum, (rather than muscular control) to achieve the posture. This lacks control, resulting in muscular damage, and could temporarily set back your steady improvement.

Stretching Tips

1. The stretching movement should be fluid, slow, restrained and controlled.

2. Never stretch beyond your comfort range. With each repetition and each session, you will steadily and easily increase your degree of stretch.

3. Concentrate! Think about each muscle as you stretch it.

4. Exercise initially in front of the mirror until you are quite sure of your alignment.

5. Hold each stretch for a count of 10. Increase the count each day if you are comfortable with the stretch.

6. Repeat each of the stretches at least three times. Since the Lunge (pages 110–112) is such an effective exercise for your outer and inner thighs, each type of lunge should be repeated five times on each side, followed by a second set on each side.

7. Many different stretches are described in this section. You should try all of them, then choose the ones that make you most invigorated and which seem to maximize your total body stretch.

8. For extra benefit, do extra stretches after the **Twelve-Minute Miracle**, the **Thigh Thinners**, and **Aerobic Exercise**.

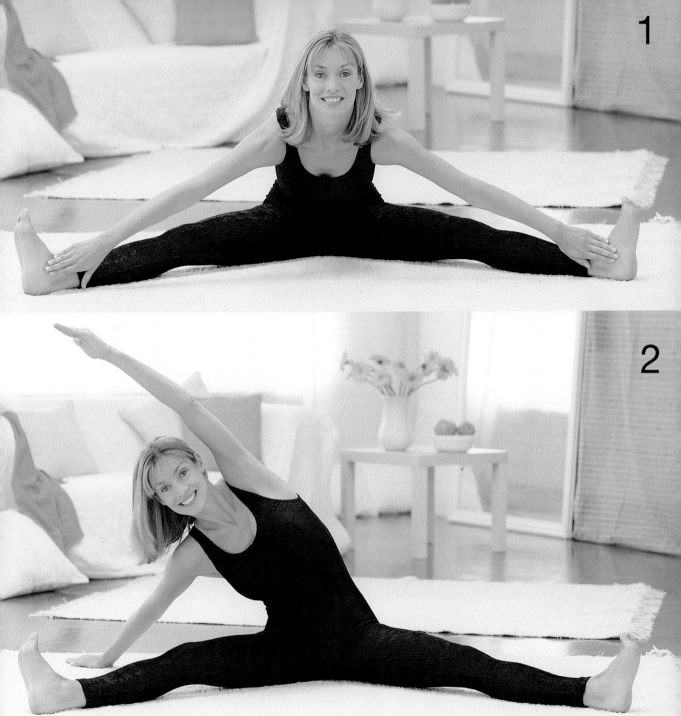

1

2

The "V"

1 Sit on the floor with your legs in as wide a "V" as possible with your ankles flexed. Keeping your back straight, lean straight forward with your arms extended to touch your inner ankles. Push your ankles as far apart as possible. Hold for a count of 20.

2 Keeping your legs in a wide "V", sit up. Place your right palm on the floor as far to the right as possible and lift your left straightened arm over your head as far to the right as possible. Push your left leg as far to the left as possible. Concentrate on the stretch in both your upper arms and your left front thigh. Hold for a count of 20.

Repeat: stretch your right arm to the left.

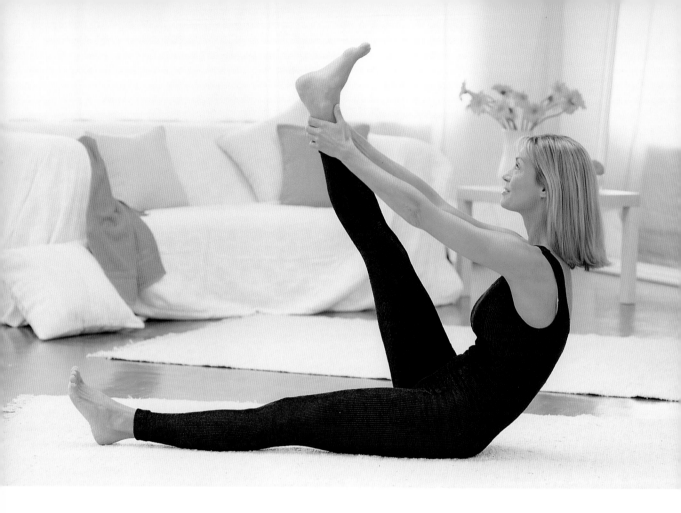

⇧ Raise the Boom I

1   Sit with your legs placed straight out in front of you with your ankles flexed.

2   Lift your right leg straight up and grasp behind your ankle with both hands. Keep your left leg straight on the floor.

3   Pull your right leg gently towards your shoulder with your hands as you push against them with your straight leg. Concentrate on the stretch at the back of your thigh.

4   Flex both feet and hold for a count of five, point both for a count of five, and flex both for a count of five.

5   Slowly lower your right leg.

Repeat: with your left leg.

⇩ Raise the Boom II

This variation of the exercise also works your abdominal muscles.

1 Lie on your back with both your legs straight out in front of you and your abdomen tightened. Start with both feet flexed.

2 Lift your right leg straight up and grasp behind your ankle with both hands. Keep your left leg straight on the floor and your back straight with your head and shoulders on the floor.

3 Pull your right leg towards your shoulder as you push against your hands with your straightened leg. Concentrate on the stretch at the back of your thigh and on your tight abdomen. Keep your back straight.

4 Flex both feet and hold for a count of five, point both for five, and flex both for five.

5 Slowly lower your right leg.

Repeat: raising your left leg.

Variation: As you become more comfortable with this stretch, keeping your back straight, raise your head and shoulders off the floor, so that you try to touch your forehead to your uplifted knee. This is excellent for tightening your abdomen.

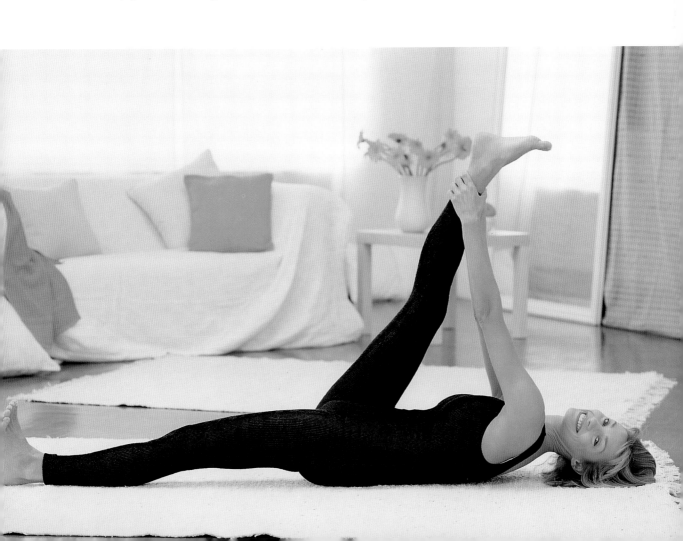

⬇ Do the Twist

1 Sit on the floor with your back straight and your legs straight out in front of you. Bend your right leg and cross your right foot over your left leg so that your right foot touches your outer left knee.

2 Straighten your right arm and press the back of your right elbow against the inside of your right knee. Keep your left leg straight and your left foot flexed.

3 Twist your torso to the left as far as you can from your waist up, putting your left hand (palm down) on the floor behind you. Turn your head to look as far over your left shoulder as possible, maximizing the stretch. Concentrate on pushing your right thigh to the left as you press the back of your elbow to the right. Hold for a count of 20.

Repeat: twisting to the other side.

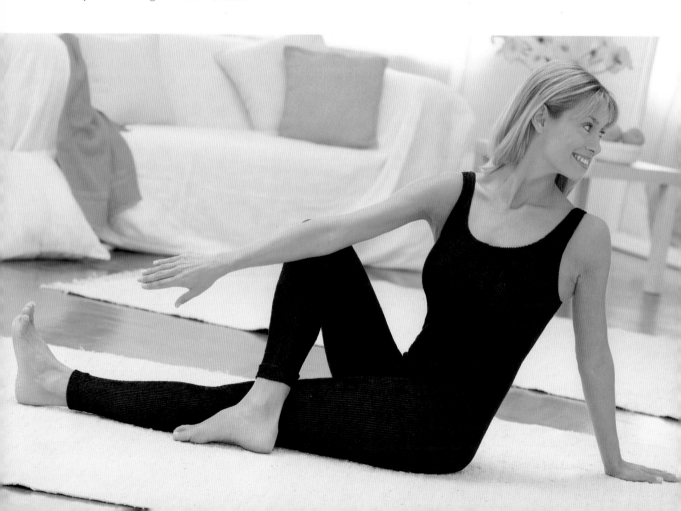

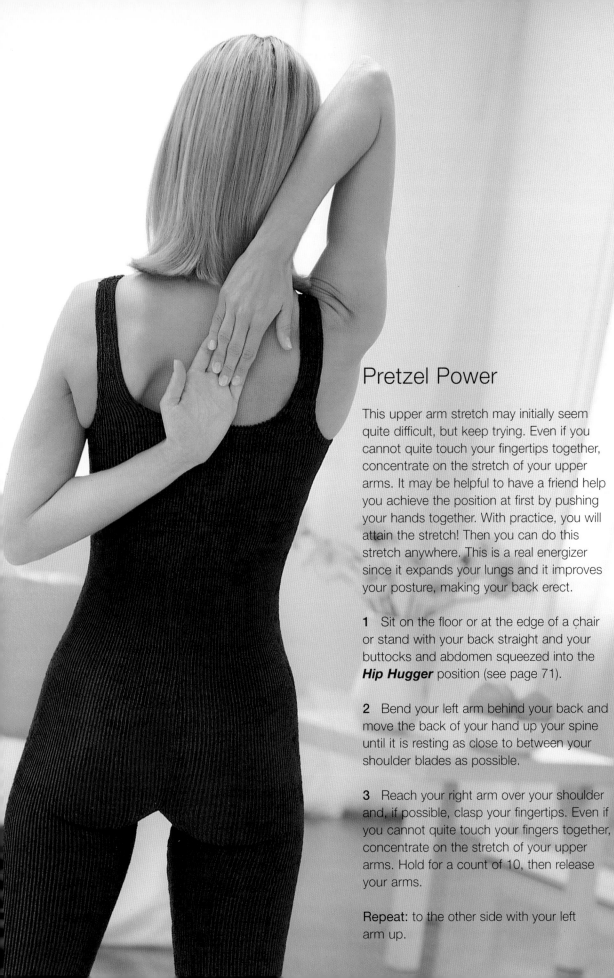

Pretzel Power

This upper arm stretch may initially seem quite difficult, but keep trying. Even if you cannot quite touch your fingertips together, concentrate on the stretch of your upper arms. It may be helpful to have a friend help you achieve the position at first by pushing your hands together. With practice, you will attain the stretch! Then you can do this stretch anywhere. This is a real energizer since it expands your lungs and it improves your posture, making your back erect.

1 Sit on the floor or at the edge of a chair or stand with your back straight and your buttocks and abdomen squeezed into the **Hip Hugger** position (see page 71).

2 Bend your left arm behind your back and move the back of your hand up your spine until it is resting as close to between your shoulder blades as possible.

3 Reach your right arm over your shoulder and, if possible, clasp your fingertips. Even if you cannot quite touch your fingers together, concentrate on the stretch of your upper arms. Hold for a count of 10, then release your arms.

Repeat: to the other side with your left arm up.

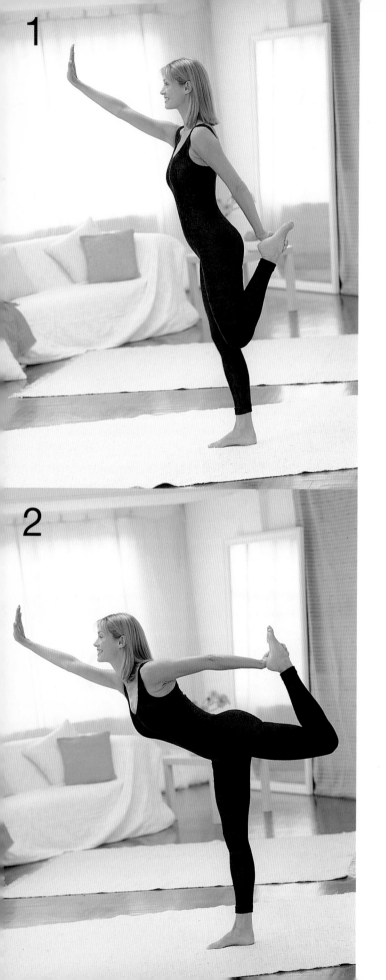

1

2

The Fountain of Youth

This stretch is quite difficult at first, but if you practise each day (holding a support if necessary), you will soon achieve this excellent total body stretch and improve your balance so that you can hold the position for up to one minute without support.

1 Stand on your right leg. Bend your left leg behind you and grasp your left inner ankle with your left hand.

2 Slowly lift your left foot, pushing your leg straight back against your hand. Try to raise your left foot behind you to the level of your shoulder. Keep your hips level and your foot pointed. As you raise your left leg, raise your right arm straight out in front of you, hand flexed, and lift it slowly toward the ceiling. Allow your gaze to follow your fingertips. Try to hold this pose for at least 10 seconds. If you have difficulty balancing at first, hold on to a bureau top or railing for support with your outstretched right hand, lifting your head to look up towards the ceiling. Concentrate on the stretch in the front of your left thigh, your upper right arm and your neck. Release.

Repeat: raising the right leg.

The Twelve Minute Miracle

This exercise routine was developed partially following the ancient therapeutic art of Hatha yoga, which improves posture and muscle tone through stretching techniques. In focusing on the muscles and correct breathing, yoga enhances concentration and increases energy. The **Twelve-Minute Miracle** is also based on ballet movements.

Why yoga and ballet? Because ballet dancers and women who practise yoga don't have cellulite! The fat responsible for the dimpled appearance of cellulite is just under the skin and over the muscle. Body-building exercises increase muscle mass, increasing the pressure on the connective tissue packages of fat so the rippled cellulite becomes more apparent. Exercises that stretch the muscles and tendons also stretch the overlying fat, so that the lumpy look disappears.

Do not feel that you don't have the flexibility or balance to attempt such lofty arts as yoga or ballet. These movements are simple and graceful. Work at your own pace. This is not meant to be a contest; you don't need to grit your teeth. There certainly is gain without pain! These exercises are peaceful and relaxing. You will be invigorated and happy after your sessions and proud of your improvement each day.

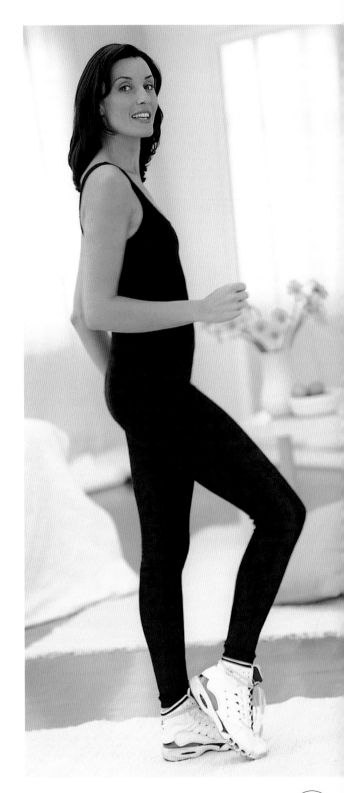

⬇ Kick 'em Out

1 Stand with your heels together and your toes turned comfortably outwards. With your left hand, hold lightly on to a waist-high support, such as a desk or the back of a steady chair.

2 With your toe pointed and your right knee out to the side, bend your right leg until your toe touches the inner side of your left knee. Keep your back straight and tighten your buttocks in the **Hip Hugger** position, pushing your right knee back as far as you comfortably can. As you practise, you will be able to increase your "turn out." Do not strain.

3 Extend your right leg straight out to the side without moving your hips (see photograph below). Slightly turn your pointed foot so that your heel subtly faces forwards. Hold this position for a count of five.

4 Now twist your right leg so that your heel subtly faces back. Hold for a count of five.

5 Flex your foot for a count of five; then point again for a count of five.

6 Bring your extended leg in again to the position in Step 2 and lift your bent (right) knee up slightly, maximizing the "turn out" of your knee, for a count of five before returning to the starting position.

Repeat: five right, five left.

Variations:
1 After turning your heel toward the wall in front of you, turn it toward the wall behind you and hold for a count of five, first with the toes pointed, then flexed, then pointed again.

2 If you feel comfortable, wear ½–2 kg (1–4 lb) ankle weights. Do not strain.

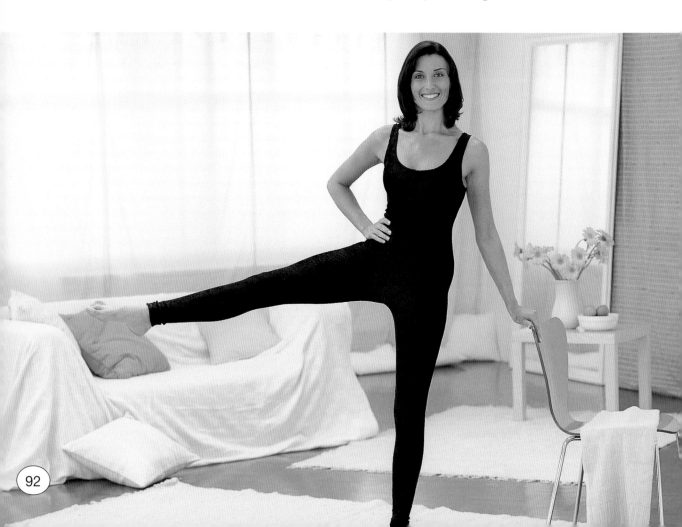

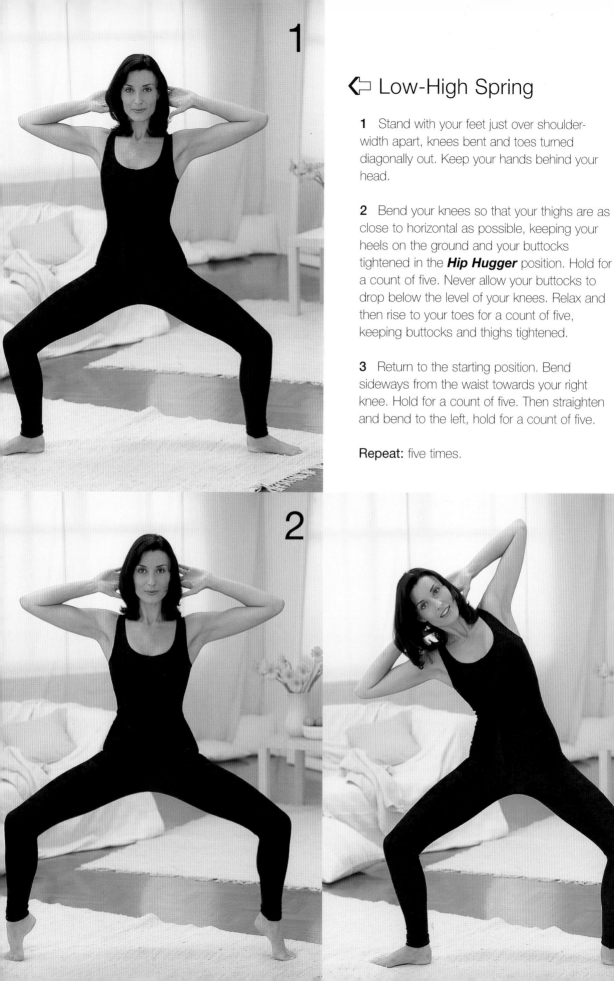

1

⬅ Low-High Spring

1 Stand with your feet just over shoulder-width apart, knees bent and toes turned diagonally out. Keep your hands behind your head.

2 Bend your knees so that your thighs are as close to horizontal as possible, keeping your heels on the ground and your buttocks tightened in the **Hip Hugger** position. Hold for a count of five. Never allow your buttocks to drop below the level of your knees. Relax and then rise to your toes for a count of five, keeping buttocks and thighs tightened.

3 Return to the starting position. Bend sideways from the waist towards your right knee. Hold for a count of five. Then straighten and bend to the left, hold for a count of five.

Repeat: five times.

2

3

⬇ Thigh-High Back Kick

1   Kneel on the floor with your knees apart, positioned under your hip bones, and your elbows straight. Keep your buttocks tight in the **Hip Hugger** contraction (see page 71); do not let your back or neck arch.

2   Lift your bent right leg behind you, forming a straight line from head to knee. Reach for the ceiling with your toe. The movement is very subtle. Hold the position for a count of five.

3   Flex your foot, reaching for the ceiling with your heel; hold for a count of five. Point your toes again: hold for a count of five.

4   Repeat with pointed toe again.

Repeat: five right, five left.

⇨ Thigh-High Side Stretch

1   Kneel on all fours on the floor with your knees apart, positioned under your hip bones, and your arms directly under your shoulders with elbows relaxed, not locked. Keep your stomach and buttocks tight in the **Hip Hugger** position (see page 71). Keeping your knee bent, lift your right leg out to the side with your thigh parallel to the floor.

2   Without moving your hips, straighten your bent leg, holding it out to the side. Actively stretch with your pointed toe.

3   Subtly twist your leg, first so that the sole of your foot turns towards the ceiling, then subtly twist so that it turns towards the floor. This twist is very effective in stretching your thigh muscles.

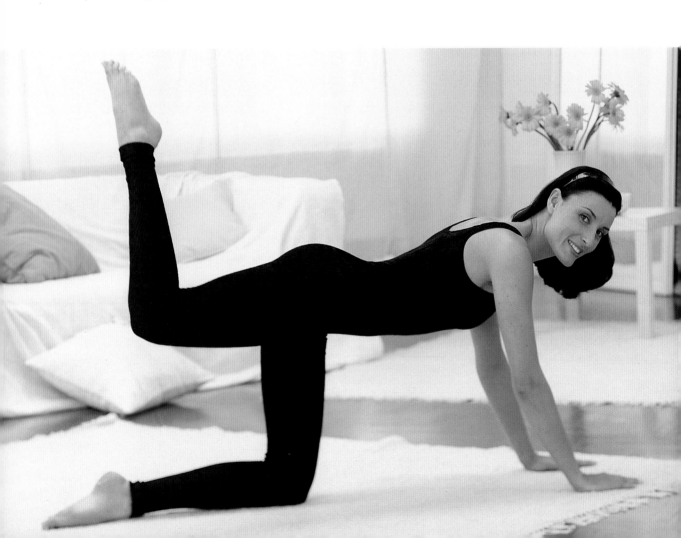

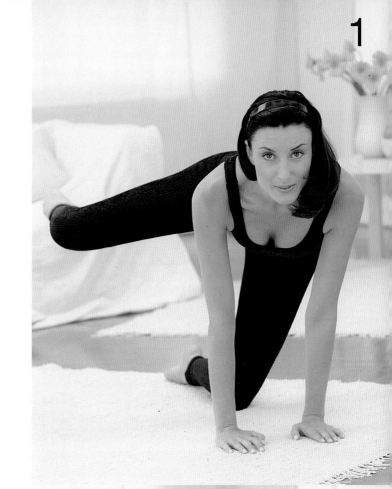

4 Repeat the stretch and twists with your foot flexed, then again with your toes pointed.

5 Return to the raised bent knee position (see photograph, right), then to the starting position.

Repeat: five right, five left.

Variation: if you feel comfortable, wear ½–2kg (1–4 lb) weights on your ankles. Do not strain.

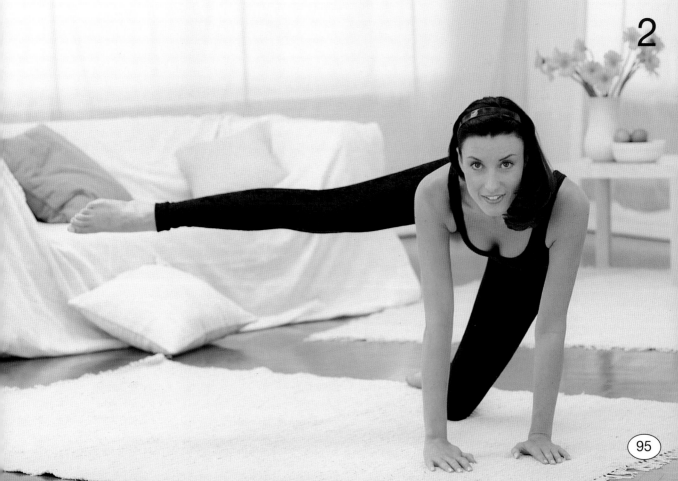

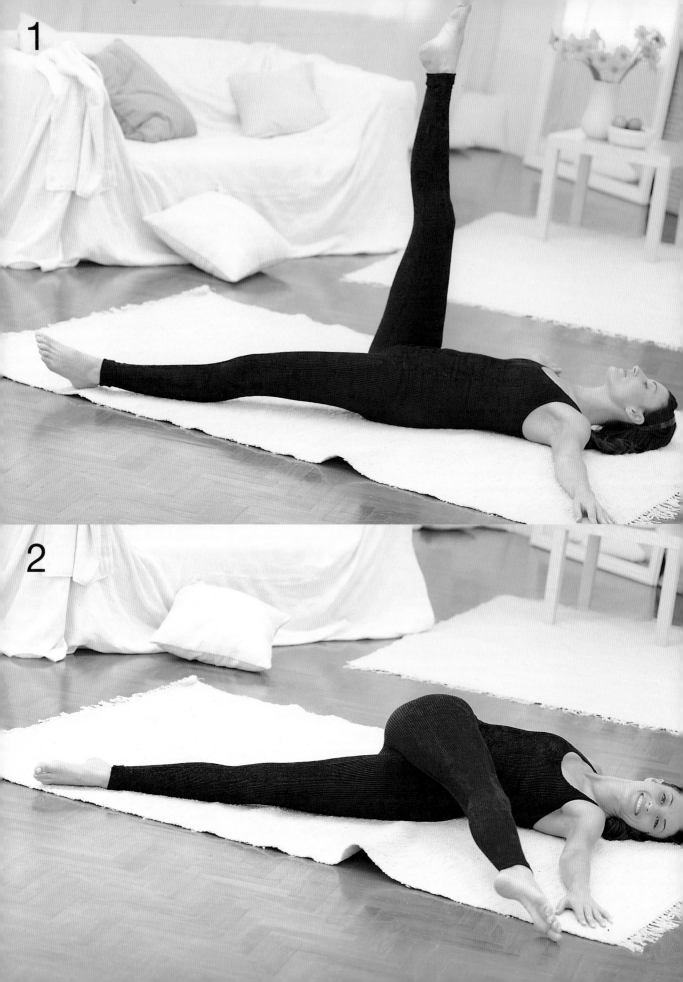

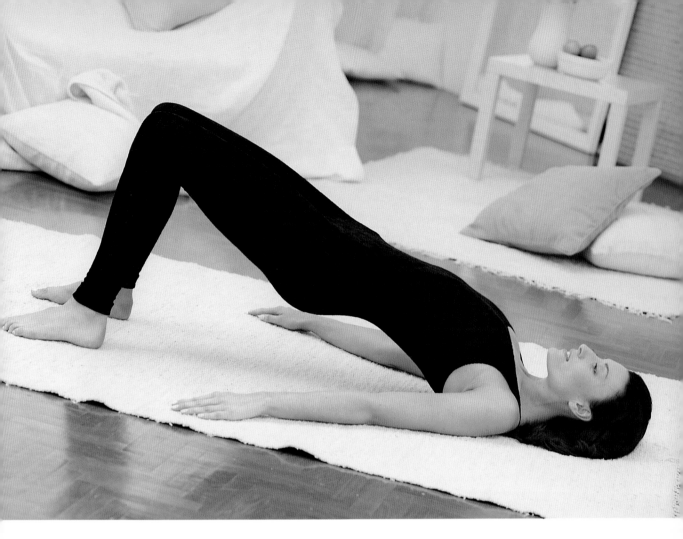

← Metronome

1 Lie on the floor on your back, with your arms stretched out to the sides and toes pointed. Lift up your right leg, pointing your toe as though you were trying to touch the ceiling. Flex your foot, and stretch as though you were trying to touch your heel to the ceiling. Again, point your toe and stretch your leg.

2 Now cross your right leg over your body to touch your left hand. Tap the floor beside your hand three times with your pointed toe, then with your heel (flexing your foot) and again with your pointed toe.

3 Return to the raised leg position in Step 1, point and flex your foot and stretch as previously, before returning to the starting position.

Repeat: five right, five left.

⬆ Bungee Buns

1 Lie on your back with your knees apart and bent and your feet flat on the floor about hip distance apart. Place your palms flat on the floor with your arms at your sides, slightly away from your body for support.

2 Lift your pelvis, forming a straight line from knees to shoulders.

3 Now tuck into the *Hip Hugger* contraction (see page 71), subtly raising your pelvis. Hold for a count of 10; release. Repeat five times.

4 In the contracted *Hip Hugger* position, bring your knees together, holding for a count of 10. You will feel the contraction in your inner thighs.

Repeat: five times.

⬇ Floor Glider

1 Lie face down, with straight legs (either together or apart) and arms stretched straight out at the sides, palms down.

2 Raise your chest and arms as high as possible. You should be looking straight ahead. Think of yourself doing a swan dive, or gliding like a svelte seagull. Hold for a count of five.

3 Lower your chest and arms and raise both legs as high as possible. Hold for a count of five.

Repeat: three times.

Variation: raise your chest, arms and legs simultaneously and hold for a count of five (see photograph, below). Do this only when it is comfortable.

1

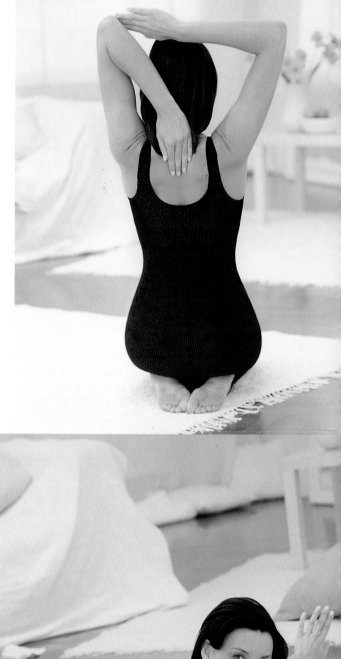

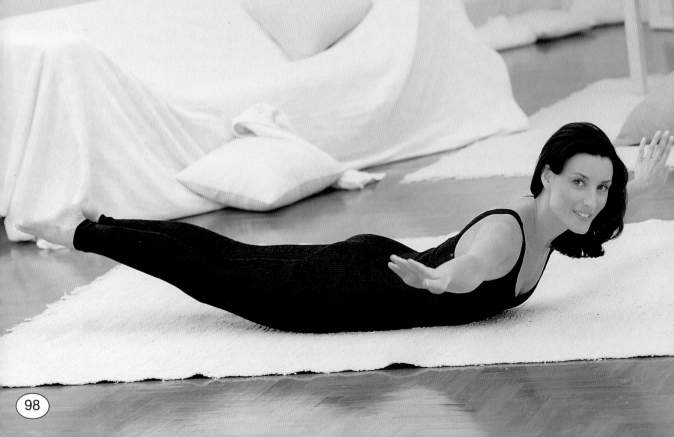

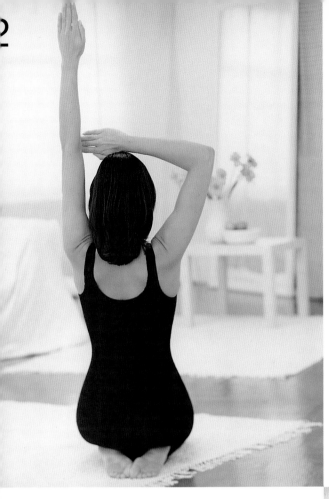

⇐ Semaphore Wave

1 Standing straight with your pelvis tucked into the *Hip Hugger* contraction (see page 71) or sitting on your feet as shown, raise your left arm straight up and bend your elbow so that your palm touches your left shoulder blade (see photograph, far left). Press your right hand with palm forward against your left elbow, pushing your elbow back for a count of 10. You will feel the stretch in the triceps.

2 Extend your left arm straight above your head, keeping your palm forward. Stretch up for a count of 10, then return to starting position.

3 Repeat Step 2 twisting your left arm so that your left palm faces back.

Repeat: five times raising your left hand, then five times raising your right hand.

⇨ Happy Hundred

1 Wearing supportive running shoes, run on the spot for 100 steps, lifting your knees high and swinging your arms. Land on the balls of your feet with bent knees, allowing your heels to touch the floor.

Variation: do jumping jacks or can-can kicks, skip or just walk briskly in place, swinging your arms and keeping your abdominal tight in the *Hip Hugger*.

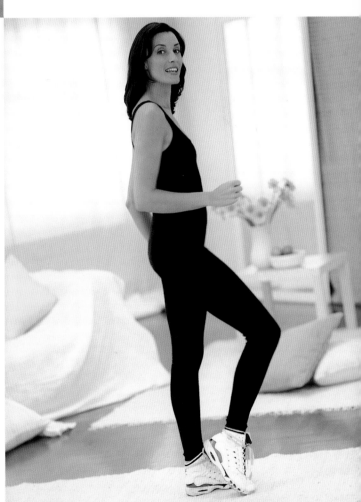

Thigh Thinners

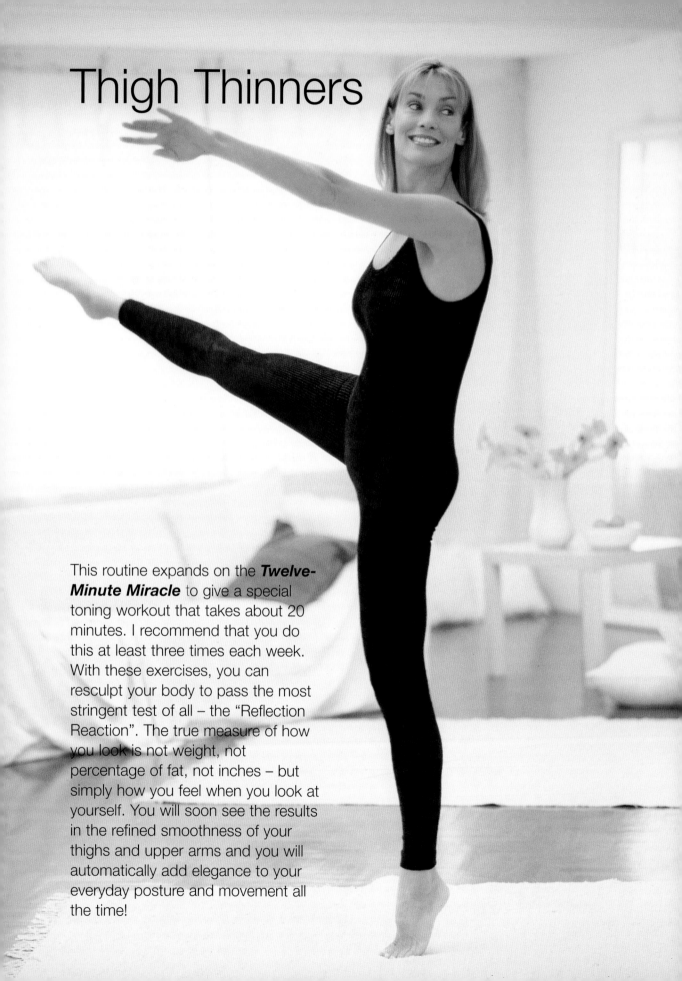

This routine expands on the **Twelve-Minute Miracle** to give a special toning workout that takes about 20 minutes. I recommend that you do this at least three times each week. With these exercises, you can resculpt your body to pass the most stringent test of all – the "Reflection Reaction". The true measure of how you look is not weight, not percentage of fat, not inches – but simply how you feel when you look at yourself. You will soon see the results in the refined smoothness of your thighs and upper arms and you will automatically add elegance to your everyday posture and movement all the time!

Laredo Low Lift

1 Lie with your right side on the floor, with your head resting on your right arm throughout this exercise. Your head, right elbow, right shoulder, hips and right ankle should remain in a straight line throughout the exercise.

2 Bend your left leg so that your left foot is flat on the floor about 2.5 cm (1 inch) in front of your hips.

3 With your right foot flexed, slowly lift your right leg off the floor as high as possible (at least half way to the height of your left shoulder). Be sure to keep your right leg straight, stretching lengthways as if trying to touch one wall of the room with your right sole and the opposite wall with your right hand.

4 Holding your right leg up, first flex your foot parallel to the floor for a count of five, then point for five, then flex again for a count of five.

5 With your leg still at the top, repeat Step 4, first flexing and pointing your foot toward the floor, then flexing and pointing your foot toward the ceiling.

6 Slowly lower your right leg to the floor with the foot flexed, concentrating on your inner thigh muscles.

Repeat: start with five right, five left; increase to 15 right, 15 left.

Variation: if you feel comfortable, wear ½–2 kg (1–4 lb) ankle weights.

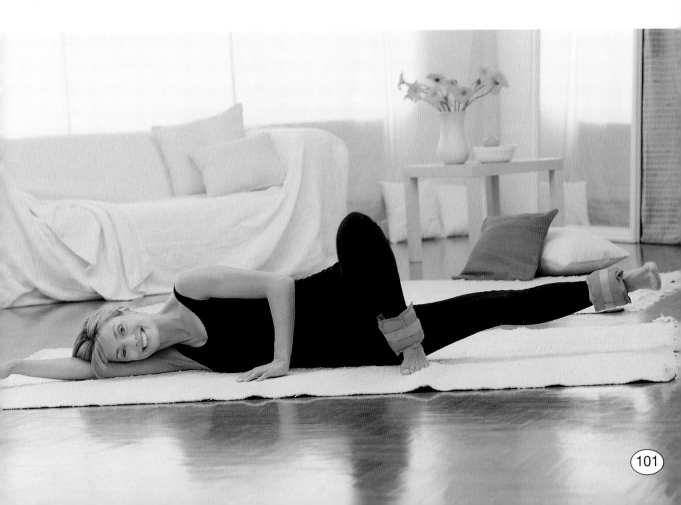

⬇ Laredo High Lift

1 Lie on your right side on the floor, with your head resting on your right arm. Your head, right elbow, right shoulder, hips and both ankles should be in a straight line.

2 Keeping your right leg straight on the floor with your foot flexed, slowly raise your left leg off the floor to the height of your left shoulder. Keep your left leg straight. Stretch both legs lengthwise as if trying to touch the wall of the room with both feet and the opposite wall with your left hand.

3 Holding your left leg up, first flex your foot parallel to the floor for a count of five, then point for a count of five, then flex again for a count of five.

4 With your leg still up, twist your ankle to point your toes toward the floor for a count of five, then flex your ankles (pointing to the floor) for a count of five. Next twist your ankle to point your toes toward the ceiling for a count of five.

5 Slowly lower your left leg to the starting position with the foot flexed, concentrating on your outer thigh muscles.

Repeat: start with five left, five right; increase to 15 left, 15 right.

Variation: if you feel comfortable, wear ½–2 kg (1–4 lb) ankle weights.

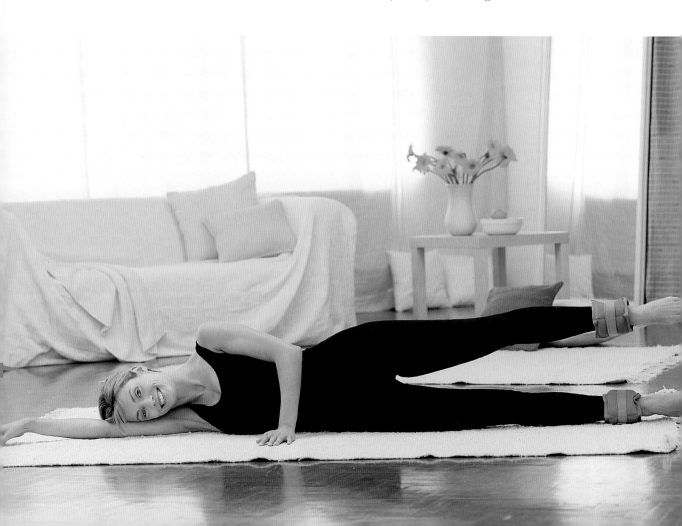

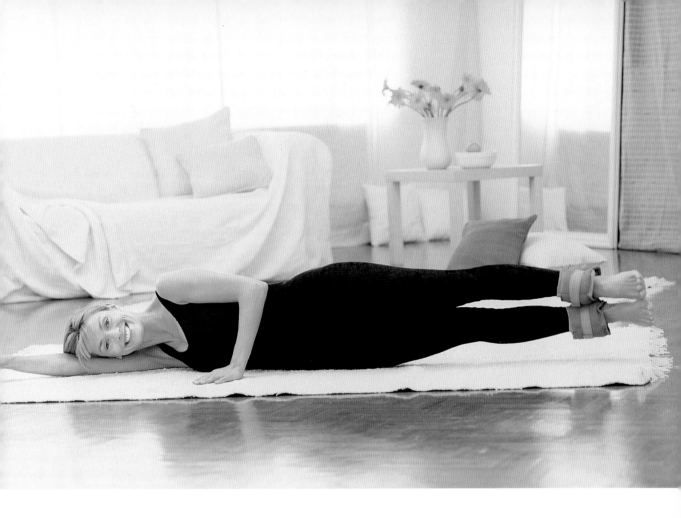

⬆ Laredo Double Lift

1 Lie on your right side on the floor, with your head resting on your right arm. Your head, right elbow, right shoulder, hips and both ankles should be in a straight line.

2 With both feet flexed, slowly lift your legs off the floor as high as possible (at least half way to the height of your left shoulder). Keep your legs straight, stretching lengthwise.

3 Holding your legs in this position, first flex your feet parallel to the floor for a count of five, then point for a count of five, then flex again for a count of five.

4 With your legs still in this position, twist your ankles to point your toes toward the floor for a count of five, then flex your ankles for a count of five. Next, twist your ankles to point

your toes toward the ceiling for a count of five, then flex for a count of five.

5 Slowly lower your legs with the feet flexed, concentrating on your inner and outer thigh muscles.

Repeat: start with five; increase to 15. Repeat, lying on your left side.

Variation: if you feel comfortable, wear ½–2 kg (1–4 lb) ankle weights.

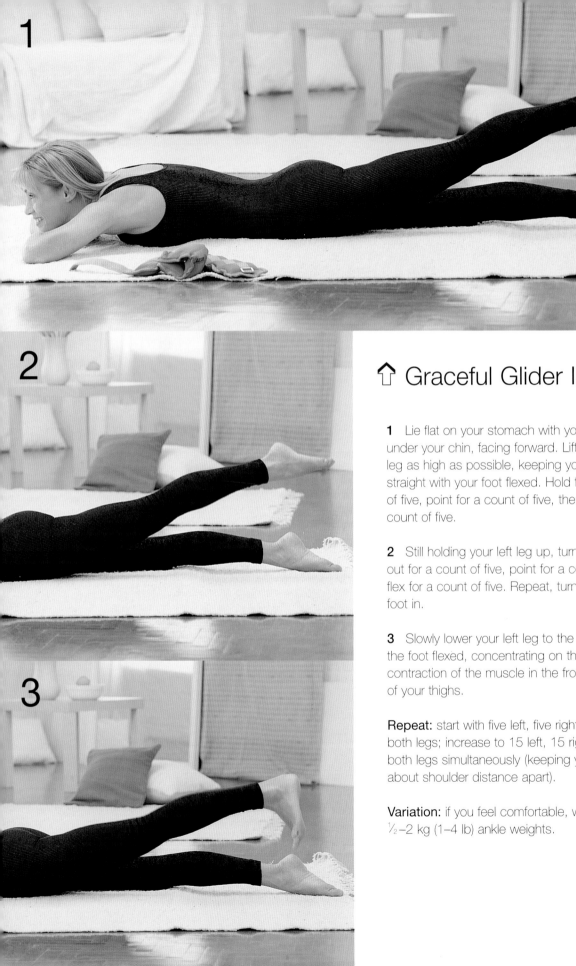

1

2

3

⇧ Graceful Glider I

1 Lie flat on your stomach with your hands under your chin, facing forward. Lift your left leg as high as possible, keeping your left leg straight with your foot flexed. Hold for a count of five, point for a count of five, then flex for a count of five.

2 Still holding your left leg up, turn your foot out for a count of five, point for a count of five, flex for a count of five. Repeat, turning your left foot in.

3 Slowly lower your left leg to the floor with the foot flexed, concentrating on the contraction of the muscle in the front and back of your thighs.

Repeat: start with five left, five right, five with both legs; increase to 15 left, 15 right, 15 with both legs simultaneously (keeping your feet about shoulder distance apart).

Variation: if you feel comfortable, wear ½–2 kg (1–4 lb) ankle weights.

⇨ Graceful Glider II

1 Lie flat on your stomach with your hands under your chin, facing forward. With your left foot flexed, bend your left knee so that your lower leg is vertical and lift as high as possible. Hold for a count of five, point for a count of five, flex for a count of five.

2 Still holding your left leg up, turn your flexed foot out for a count of five, point for a count of five, flex for a count of five. Repeat, turning your left foot in.

3 Slowly lower your left leg to the floor with the foot flexed, concentrating on the muscle contraction in the front and back of the thighs.

Repeat: start with five left, five right, five with both legs; increase to 15 left, 15 right, 15 with both legs (keeping feet shoulder distance apart).

Variation: if you feel comfortable, wear 1–4 lb (½–2 kg) ankle weights.

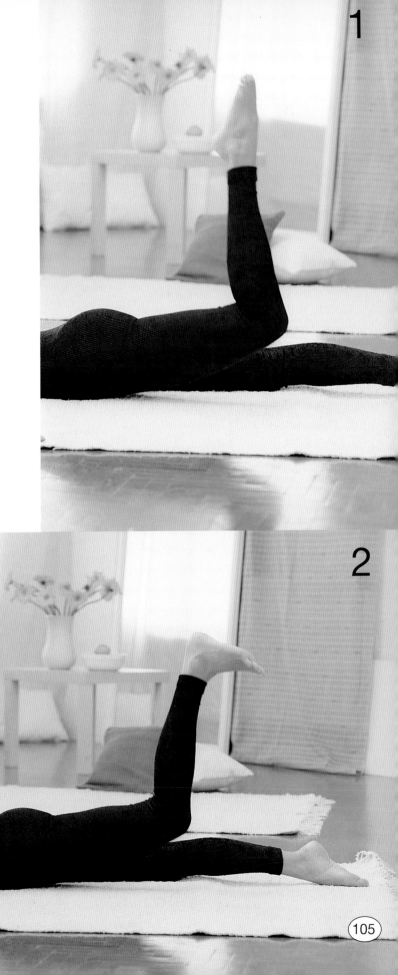

1

2

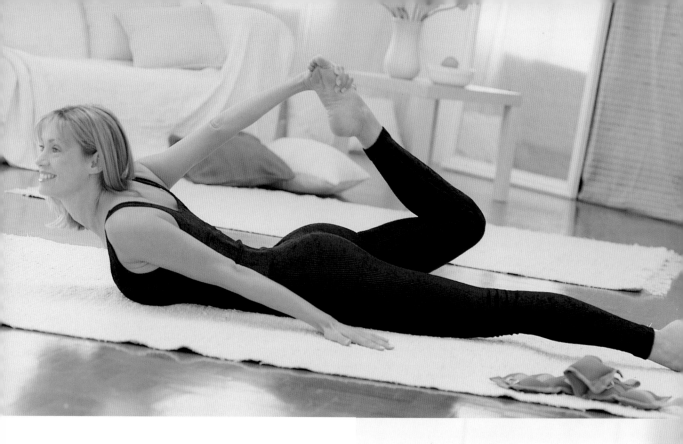

⇧ Rocking Horse

This is a total body toner!

Caution: if you have back problems, check with your doctor before doing this exercise.

1 Lie on your stomach with your head lifted, facing forward and your arms in front of you. Keeping both feet flexed, grasp your right foot with your right hand, lifting your torso and chin as far as you can.

2 Lift your right thigh as high and as far as possible. Hold with your foot flexed for a count of five, then point for a count of five, then flex for a count of five. Concentrate on the stretch of your upper arm, thigh and chin.

3 Slowly return to the starting position.

Repeat: start with five right, five left, five with both legs (see photograph, right); increase to 15 right, 15 left, 15 with both legs.

Variation: if you feel comfortable, wear ½–2 kg (1–4 lb) ankle weights.

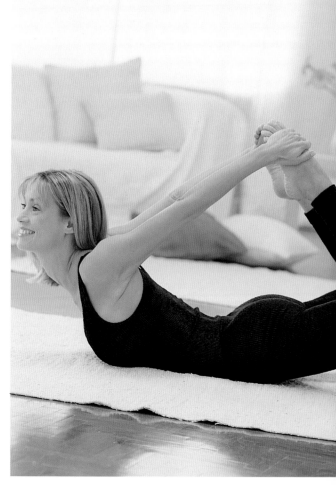

➡️ Air Scissor

This fabulous excercise helps your stomach as well as your thighs!

1 Prop yourself up on your left elbow, lifting both legs to the ceiling. Grasp your right ankle with your right hand, putting your leg as close to your shoulder as possible, keeping your right arm and right leg straight.

2 Place your left leg next to your right leg, then scissor first out to the left side so that your left leg touches the floor. Keep both feet flexed for a count of five, then point for a count of five, and flex again for a count of five.

3 Slowly scissor your left leg upward and inward, positioning it in front of your uplifted right leg as far as possible with both feet flexed, concentrating on your inner thigh muscle. Hold in that position for a count of five, then point both feet for a count of five, and finally flex for a count of five.

4 Slowly lower your left leg to the floor.

5 Slowly scissor your left leg upward and inward but position it behind your uplifted right leg as far as possible with both feet flexed for a count of five, then point both for a count of five, and then flex again for a count of five. Lower your left leg to the floor.

Repeat: start with five left, five right; increase to 15 left, 15 right.

Variation: if you feel comfortable, wear ½-2 kg (1–4 lb) ankle weights. You may prefer to do this exercise propped on both elbows, making the right scissor easier. Be sure to stretch your uplifted right leg towards your shoulder!

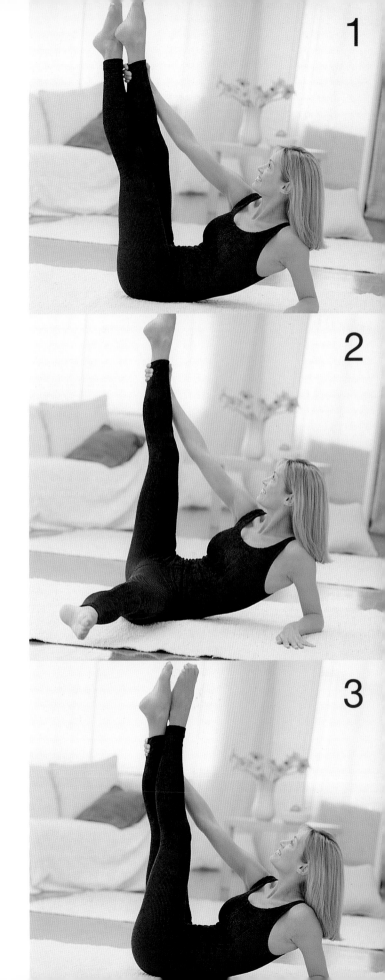

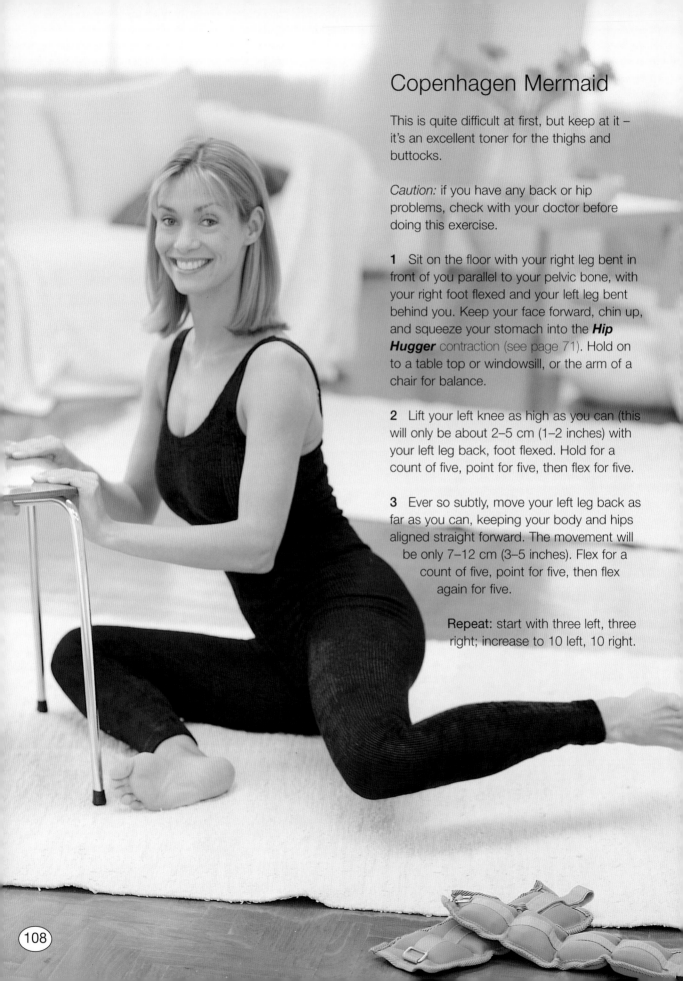

Copenhagen Mermaid

This is quite difficult at first, but keep at it – it's an excellent toner for the thighs and buttocks.

Caution: if you have any back or hip problems, check with your doctor before doing this exercise.

1   Sit on the floor with your right leg bent in front of you parallel to your pelvic bone, with your right foot flexed and your left leg bent behind you. Keep your face forward, chin up, and squeeze your stomach into the **Hip Hugger** contraction (see page 71). Hold on to a table top or windowsill, or the arm of a chair for balance.

2   Lift your left knee as high as you can (this will only be about 2–5 cm (1–2 inches) with your left leg back, foot flexed. Hold for a count of five, point for five, then flex for five.

3   Ever so subtly, move your left leg back as far as you can, keeping your body and hips aligned straight forward. The movement will be only 7–12 cm (3–5 inches). Flex for a count of five, point for five, then flex again for five.

Repeat: start with three left, three right; increase to 10 left, 10 right.

Air Seat

1 Stand with feet parallel, straight ahead, about shoulder width apart. Rest your hands on your back waist, with your palms out and fingers intertwined. Keep your arms and shoulders back as far as possible and pull your abdomen into the **Hip Hugger** position (see page 71). Keep your back straight.

2 Squat down as though you are about to sit in a chair. Concentrate on squeezing your thighs and buttocks together and pushing your shoulders back. Hold for a count of five and resume starting position. (Your rear end will go out and your shoulders will move forward.)

Repeat: start with five; increase to 10.

Variation: start with your hands on your hips. Raise your hands to the front as you hold the squat to maintain balance (see photograph, below right). You may wish to wear ½–1½ kg (1–3 lb) wrist weights.

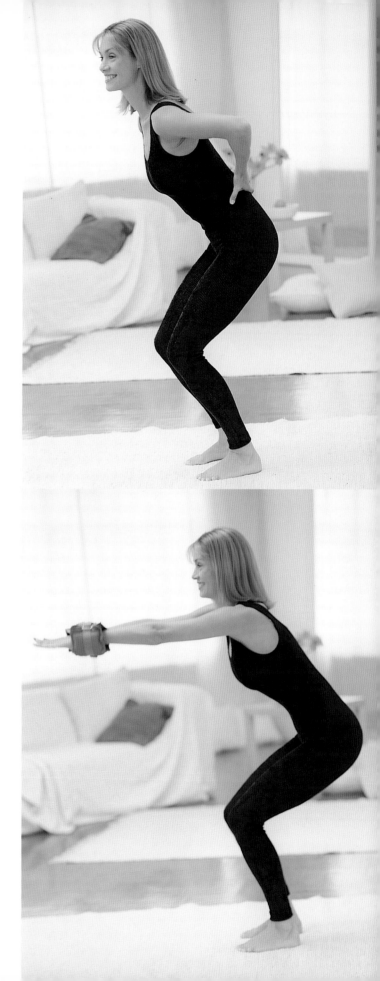

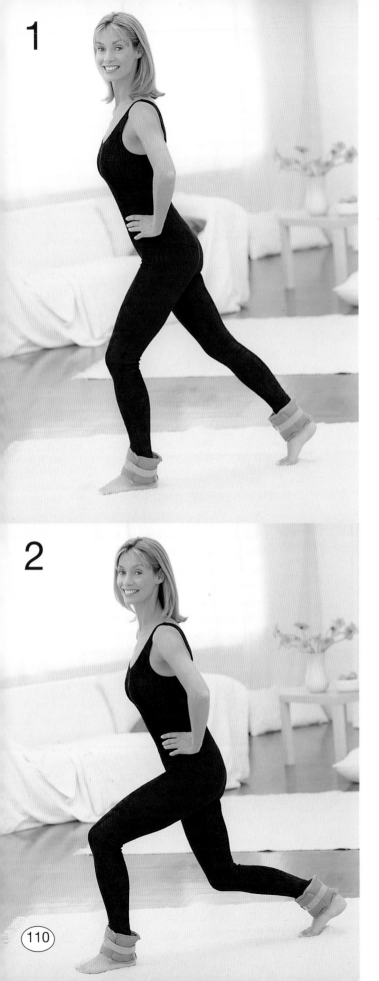

1

2

The Lunge

The lunge is one of the best exercises for shaping the thighs and buttocks, as well as helping posture and balance. The trick is to do it properly.

⇦ Forward Stride

1 Start with your feet about shoulder-width apart. Step your left leg forward about 90 cm (3 feet), placing your heel down first.

2 Keeping your spine straight, lower yourself so that your front left knee bends to a 90° angle with your knee over your ankle. Your back right leg will also be bent to a 90° angle with the ankle flexed.

3 Step forward to the starting position, pressing your heel into the floor as you lift.

4 Step forward with your right foot.

Repeat: start with10 full steps forward (right and left); increase to 30 full steps forward.

Backward Stride ⇨

1 Start with your feet about shoulder-width apart. Then lift your left leg and step back 60 cm (2 feet).

2 Keeping your spine straight, lower yourself so that your forward right knee bends to a 90° angle with your knee over your ankle. Your back left knee should also be bent to 90° with your ankle flexed.

3 To return to the starting position, press your weight into the front heel for balance and then step backward.

4 Step backward with your right leg.

Repeat: start with 10 full steps backward (right and left); increase to 30 full steps backward.

⇨ Superhero Lunge

1 Stand with back and neck straight, with your pelvis in the *Hip Hugger* position. Step forward about 76 cm (2½ ft) with your right leg, turning your left foot out, and keeping your right foot straight so that your feet form a 90-degree angle. Transfer your weight forward onto the right leg. With your heel pressed down, your right knee should be directly above, never in front of your ankle. As you improve, your right thigh will be lower, parallel to the floor. You will feel the contraction on the outer thigh (the quadriceps) of the forward leg and the stretch on the inner thigh (the adductor) of the straightened leg. Hold for a count of 10.

2 Keeping the same stance, relax, turn your left foot so that it faces forward. Keeping your leg straight and lifting your left heel off the floor, stretch the left quadriceps. Hold for a count of 10. The greater the distance between your feet, the better the stretch on your straight, back leg. Increase the length of the stance as

much as you can each day without straining. Keep your back straight at all times.

Repeat: five left, five right.

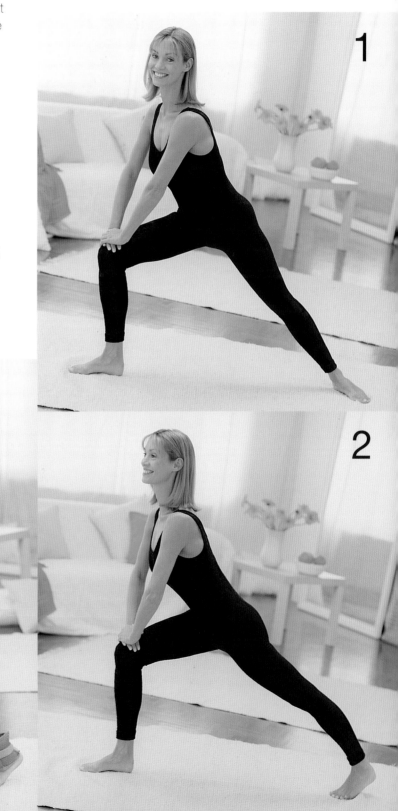

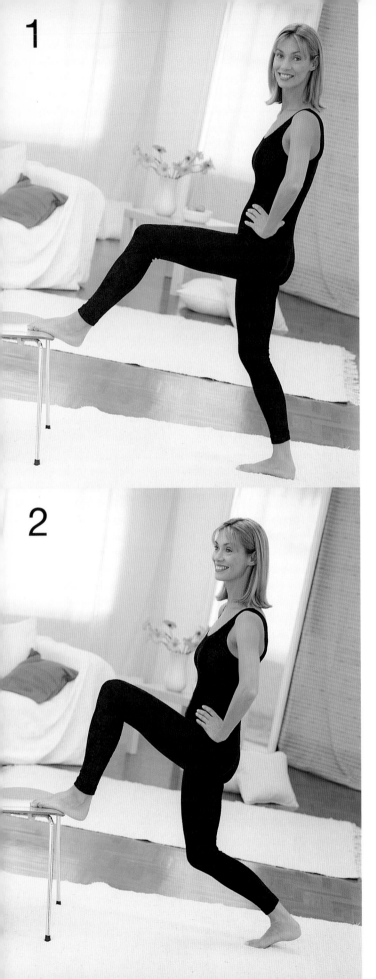

1

2

⬅ Step-Up Stride

Lunging on to a 20 cm (8 inch) platform really works the buttocks and the backs of the thighs.

1 Stand 60–90 cm (2–3 feet) behind a platform (such as a firm chair or bench or sofa) and step forward on to it, keeping your heel down.

2 Keeping your spine straight, lower yourself so that your front leg bends to a 90° angle with your knee over your ankle.

3 Return to your starting position by pressing your heel into the platform as you straighten up.

Repeat: start with 10 steps-ups to each side; increase to 30 step-ups.

Variation: hold 1½–4 kg (3–8 lb) weights in your hands, keeping your arms extended to the side.

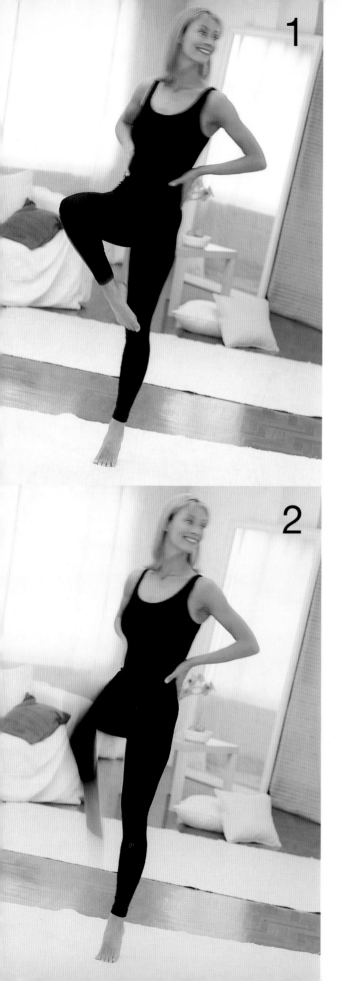

⬅ Can-Can

Pretend you are a Rockette at Radio City Music Hall in New York! Dance with joy!

1   Put your hands on your hips, look to the left. Kick up your right leg, bending your knee to touch your right foot on your left knee. Return to starting position.

2   Then kick up your right leg as high as you can straight in front of you, pointing your toe. (See also page 100.) Lower to the starting position.

3   Kick your right leg, bending your knee to touch your right foot to your left knee again.

4   Kick your right leg as high as you can to the right side.

Repeat: 50 kicks to each side.

Variation: create a swimming motion by touching your left hand to your right ankle as you kick your right leg up, lifting your right arm to your right side.

Aerobic Exercise

Think how children move and play: running, jumping, climbing, using their whole bodies. They show the flexibility and range of motion and energy that we all once had. As adults, we move slowly and deliberately – and barely at all! Most of us just sit for hours each day in offices, in cars, in front of television or at meals. We take the lift instead of climbing stairs. We drive even short distances, rather than walk.

All of the conveniences of today's life encourage inactivity. Our grandparents chopped wood for the stove instead of putting food into the microwave; people worked in the fields; now they sit in front of computers, working only their mouse; we even shop by mail order and control our televisions by remote control rather than crossing the room to switch the button.

We are suffering from a serious epidemic of inactivity. The frightening reality in America is that 25 per cent of the adult population does 80 per cent of the exercise! The other 75 per cent are at risk of all of the health problems associated with inactivity. About half of us don't even get enough exercise to raise our heart rates above "idle". One-quarter of all Americans do no exercise at all!

Laziness is hazardous to your health

Steven N. Blair, P.E.D., of the Cooper Institute for Aerobics Research in Dallas believes that inactivity is "as important as any public health problem we have". It has been estimated that about 150,000 people a year die as a result of inactivity: a sedentary lifestyle is almost as serious a health risk as smoking cigarettes or driving after drinking alcohol.

The best way to lose extra fat is with aerobic exercise. Aerobic exercise uses stored fat from all over the body (subcutaneous fat as well as the fat that cushions the organs and the tiny strands of fat between muscle fibres) as fuel, just as a fire uses oxygen to burn coal or wood.

Fat is a dense fuel: sugar contains 4 kcals of energy per gram; fat contains 9 kcals per gram! That's why fatty foods are fattening. They give more kcals of energy, but if that energy is not used, it is stored as fat!

Aerobic Tips

1 Aerobic exercise does not require that a person be out of breath or exhausted – in fact, quite the contrary – but it must be of long enough duration (at least 30 minutes three times each week) to have the desired effect.

2 The optimal intensity of aerobic exercise is such that your heart rate should be 70 to 85 per cent of your own maximal heart rate (beats per minute or BPM). This is high enough to give an effective workout, yet low enough for you to sustain it for 20–40 minutes.

Maximal heart rate (BPM) = 220 – age (in years)
Optimal exercise heart rate
(BPM) = (0.70 to 0.85) x maximal heart rate

3 Never push yourself too hard! Even if you do not achieve 70 per cent of your maximal heart rate at first, just do the exercise continuously at your own pace for at least 20 minutes. You can increase the pace and the duration slightly each day.

4 Exercise to music you enjoy or in front of the television to energize you and to prevent boredom. Increasing the music's tempo week by week motivates you to increase the pace without straining yourself.

5 Choose an aerobic activity that is convenient and fun!

The Benefits of Aerobic Exercise to Health

1 Fat is burned.

2 Cardiovascular fitness is increased. The heart muscle becomes stronger and pumps more blood with each stroke. With this increased efficiency, the heart beats more slowly when you are inactive, but with exercise gives an even greater increase in oxygenation with each stroke, so you can exercise more intensely and for longer.

3 Aerobic exercise helps the skeletal system. Joints become more flexible with a fuller range of motion, and the bones are strengthened by improved bone remodelling. (Exercise even increases bone mineral content in post-menopausal women.)

4 Exercise may decrease the risk of certain kinds of cancer. There is evidence to suggest that even moderate aerobic exercise (such as walking only 3 km (2 miles) in 30 to 40 minutes each day, 6 days per week) decreases not only the overall death rate and the number of deaths due to heart disease, but also the number of deaths due to cancer.

5 Aerobic exercise raises the basal metabolic rate (BMR). This means that the body burns more kcals for every activity, even resting. This is in contrast to dieting which decreases the BMR: when given less food, the body conserves its use of energy, in preparation for famine. On the other hand, exercise maintains and builds muscle, thereby maintaining or increasing the BMR. Muscle burns 37.5 times more kcals than the same weight of fat: 0.4 kg (1 lb) of fat requires only 2 kcals per day, whereas 0.4 kg (1 lb) of muscle requires 75 kcals per day. Aerobic exercise really does change your body composition: fat is reduced and muscle is increased.

6 Exercise decreases appetite. The good news is that the more sedentary and overweight a person is, the more appetite will decrease with movement. "If it weren't for the fact that the TV set and the refrigerator are so far apart, some of us wouldn't get any exercise at all," says the New York humorist Joey Adams. So, instead of heading for the refrigerator immediately whenever you start to feel hungry, force yourself to do just 10 or 20 minutes of aerobic movement first. Maybe you won't even want that snack! Try exercising regularly before meals to suppress appetite.

7 Exercise really does give tone and definition where there might otherwise be "flab"! Exercise always makes you look better, even if you gain a little weight in replacing light fat with denser muscle.

8 Exercise exhilarates. It is a natural anti-depressant! Even mild exercise stimulates the production and release of endorphins, the body's own pleasure opiates. Trained athletes often describe feeling "high". Endorphins have been shown to control appetite and to reduce anxiety. Perhaps due to endorphin release, exercise wards off depression, often a cause of overeating. The more you exercise, the more you can exercise and the more you want to exercise - a great positive cycle.

Your Daily Life

There are two ways in which you can easily incorporate aerobic exercise into your daily life without impinging on your schedule at all. First never drive when you can walk or climb. Walk to work, or at least walk part of the way, getting off the bus or train one stop early. Make some of your errands an exercise outing by either walking to the stores or parking your car a short distance from the entrance. Walk up stairs instead of just waiting for the lift or do **Pressometrics** as you wait. Second, make an effort to move a bit faster than your natural pace. Burn a few more kcals with a little more action!

These seemingly minor increases in exercise really add up, especially if you increase your activity incrementally each day. If your weight is 64 kg (140 lb), by walking for 10 minutes extra each day and climbing only four flights of stairs (not necessarily at the same time!), you burn at least 17,500 kcals each year. You could lose 2.3 kg (5 lb) instead of gaining the annual average of 0.4 kg (1 lb) from inactivity. As you now realize, healthy eating helps, but for good health and permanent weight control, aerobic exercise is the key. And the results are absolutely immediate!

Types of Aerobic Exercise

Walking

Walking is the best exercise – especially for anyone who has not been active, and for busy individuals who do not have time to change clothes for jogging, to warm up and to shower. Anyone can go for a walk (even in office clothes) by simply keeping their walking shoes always available. You can walk anywhere, anytime. You do not need a treadmill or a track! You can walk outside for the fun of experiencing new scenes and getting fresh air. You can walk on the spot at home while watching television or with music to set your pace. You can walk alone to meditate, or you can walk at a planned time with a friend.

For maximum benefit:

1 Walk with a long stride.
2 Actively swing your arms like a pendulum with each step.
3 Place the heel of your leading foot down before the toe. After you have increased your pace comfortably, you may want to add 450 g (1 lb) wrist weights, or just carry a can of soup in each hand.
4 Walk "tight" - keep your abdomen and hips contracted in the **Hip Hugger** as you walk.

Jogging

Many people do the "in" exercise of the decade: jogging. Recently, however, orthopaedists and exercise physiologists have discovered that jogging can cause injuries to knees, legs, and backs. My advice to confirmed joggers is to jog only where there is fresh air (not in the pollution of traffic or industry), to wear good supportive shoes, to jog on a soft surface (not concrete), and to be moderate, not compulsive. I recommend fast walking instead of jogging since there is less danger of injury due to impact, and walking can burn as many kcals as jogging. (Walking 3 km (2 miles) in 30 minutes burns the same number of extra kcals as jogging 1.5 km (1 mile) in 10 minutes.)

Skipping

Skipping is as effective as jogging for burning kcals and has the advantage that it can be done indoors or out. If you don't have a skipping rope, an old clothesline or extension cord (not plugged in!) and well-padded shoes are all you need. Since even the lowest rate requires a lot of energy, jump for two to three minute periods, walking on the spot in between. Music really helps. Be sure to jump on the balls of your feet and to alternate feet in a skipping action; do not jump with both feet at the same time.

Climbing Steps

Walking up stairs exercises the entire body. If you work or live on an upper floor, this is an ideal exercise. Take it at your own speed.

Even if you walk halfway, you gain by climbing the first few flights. Walking upstairs is far better than using an expensive, indoor step machine. You burn fewer kcals on a machine since you need not pick up your feet and you may lean on the rails. If you do not have steps in your home or in your office, just step up and down on a thick book, preferably to music. If you have knee problems, don't climb stairs for fitness unless you consult your doctor first.

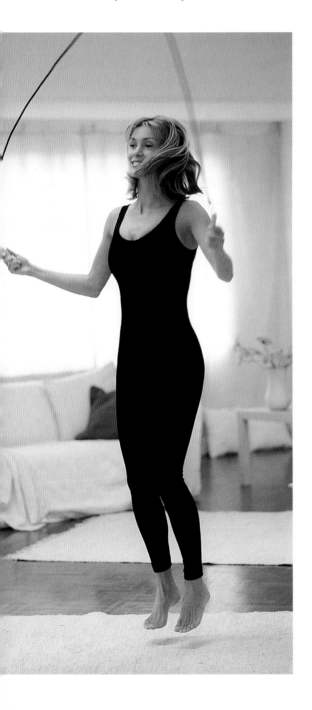

Swimming

Your can swim at any age, even when other activities might be limited by injury or by diseases such as arthritis. Swimming uses your whole body and is impact free; there is no stress on joints. Water-resistance increases the intensity of any workout. To maximize the benefits, think about your thigh and arm muscles with each stroke, contracting your thighs as you kick. Cup your hands or hold small paddles to increase resistance and maximize exercise. You need not limit yourself to swimming laps. You can walk vigorously across the pool in shoulder-high water; and you can do kicks and stretches while holding on to the side.

Rebounding

A rebounder is a springy mat like a miniature trampoline except that the fabric and construction are designed for only a little spring (not to catapult acrobats into the air). A rebounder is not expensive and it allows you to do all aerobic jumping (jogging, jumping jacks, hopping, kicking) without the danger of impact injuries. The kcals burned depend upon the activity. Rebounding exercise is an especially good way for a sedentary person to begin exercising. It is even possible for an elderly person or an invalid to benefit by bouncing the hips in a sitting position, or to exercise the legs alone with someone else jumping. People with difficulty in balance should not use the rebounder. Take it slowly at the beginning, and be careful.

Extra kcals burned in 30 minutes of exercise if you weigh 64 kg (140 lb)

Skipping	286 kcals
Jogging	286 kcals
Playing ball	160 kcals
Golf	128 kcals
Kite flying	100 kcals
Yoga	96 kcals
Rebounding	80 kcals

From the Skin In

Cellulite may originate beneath the skin, but its unattractive appearance is very much on the surface! Fortunately, simple surface treatment can not only make your skin look smoother and healthier, but can also decrease the cellulite underneath. Let's learn about three easy systems:

- skin brushing
- exfoliation
- massage

These techniques are no substitute for maintaining the right body weight and toning your muscles, but if you spend a little time each day following these skin care routines, they will definitely help you look better. They will complement the improvement that you will already have achieved through eating properly and exercising regularly, and they'll help keep your body smooth and free from cellulite.

SKIN BRUSHING

Skin brushing has been used in skin care for centuries. In many parts of the world – notably Japan and Sweden – skin brushing is a part of a woman's daily beauty and hygiene routine. Now this technique is increasingly popular in many parts of Europe and America. Dry skin brushing enhances the health and appearance of the skin by:

- removing dead skin cells which stick to the outer layer making the skin surface rough and dry.
- polishing the skin to give a youthful, silky smoothness.
- accelerating the turnover of skin cells and connective tissue so that the surface of the skin is renewed and the collagen sacks are remodelled more rapidly.

- improving the circulation within the enormous network of capillaries which lie within the deep layers of skin and in the subcutaneous fat.
- improving the lymphatic flow.

The Technique

What to use? First of all, give yourself the gift of a massage glove with stiff, densely spaced natural bristles. Brush your entire body, beginning with the tips of the extremities and moving to the centre of the body in this order:

- feet
- legs
- calves
- thighs
- buttocks
- lower back
- stomach
- sides
- hands
- arms
- shoulders
- upper back

Concentrate on the areas where your cellulite is worst. Brush your inner and outer thighs and buttocks, several times. Don't forget to brush the areas that are more difficult to reach such as just below your buttocks and just above your knees. To prevent missing important spots, brush in front of a mirror.

How hard?

Brush firmly, so you feel invigorated, but do not brush too strongly – you don't want to hurt yourself! You should have a warm pink glow afterwards, not irritated, red skin. Never brush any areas where the skin is cut or inflamed or where you have a rash.

In what direction?

You may find it more comfortable to brush standing. Raise the leg you are brushing up on to a stool or the side of the bath. Always brush in the direction from the tips of the extremities to the top of the leg or arm, following the return blood flow towards the heart.

Brush with long sweeps on the legs and arms and with rounded, half-circle motions on the thighs, stomach and back.

How often?
The best strategy is to brush the skin twice a day – in the morning when you get up (before your bath or shower) and again at night just before you go to bed.

For how long?
You can brush your entire body in less than 5 minutes. If you're short of time, even 1 or 2 minutes, concentrating on the cellulite prone areas of your body, will make a noticeable difference.

EXFOLIATION

Some of the benefits of skin brushing can also be achieved by using an exfoliant designed to remove the thick layers of dead surface skin cells. After extensive research, I have formulated a unique exfoliant for my exclusive *Longévité*® skin care products, which gently sticks to dead surface cells to peel them off. This exfoliant can even be used safely on the face, where it smoothes small wrinkles and reduces enlarged pores. Exfoliants with sandy grains must always be used with caution, particularly on the face where the particles can get into the eyes; however, they are appropriate for the areas of the body prone to cellulite, such as the thighs, back and upper arms. Exfoliate your body using the same movements as in skin brushing.

Exfoliate once or twice a day, before your bath or shower. It should take less than 5 minutes. As with skin brushing – even 1 or 2 minutes each time, concentrating on the cellulite prone areas of your body, will make a difference.

MASSAGE

Massage is one of the most relaxing and enjoyable treatments for the problem of cellulite. The physical movements in massage actually manipulate the fat tissue under the skin, improving both circulation and lymphatic drainage even more effectively than skin brushing. Increased blood circulation automatically mitigates the adverse effect of little valves within the tiny blood vessels which would otherwise constrict to aggravate the appearance of cellulite.

But no matter how beneficial massage might be, it does not – and cannot – "dissolve" fat! Massage is therefore of little value in eliminating cellulite unless it is combined with weight loss (when appropriate) and with toning exercises. There are many beauty salons and health clinics which offer so-called specialized cellulite massage, usually combined with the application of special lotions or oils. These professional treatments are usually expensive, yet they offer nothing that you cannot do for yourself at home.

Self-massage
As with skin brushing, it is a good idea to massage in front of a mirror so you can be quite sure that you treat all areas of your body that suffer from cellulite. The massage strokes should be firm but not so hard that they cause pain or bruising. Always direct massage strokes towards the heart, as described for skin brushing. I recommend that you massage once or twice a day, just after skin brushing.

What to do
Before you begin to massage any particular area of the body, apply a lotion, gel or oil of your choice. This will help your hands glide smoothly over your skin.

There are currently many new and expensive toning and anti-cellulite gels and lotions which promise "complex action to slim, firm, and tighten" for "sensational body contouring". There is considerable controversy, however, as to the efficacy of these products compared with much less expensive lotions and potions.

Some of these so-called anti-cellulite products contain esoteric ingredients from plants and algae (of possible though questionable efficacy). Others have components which have been proven to be effective on isolated fat cells. These scientifically studied ingredients are – believe it or not – caffeine and the structurally similar molecules theophyllin and aminophyllin. When caffeine is added to fat cells in the laboratory, it acts on specific enzymes to decrease the storage of fat in two ways: by inhibiting the transport of fat into fat cells and by breaking down the stored fat within fat cells. One application is equivalent to drinking less than half a cup of coffee. Whether the caffeine is delivered effectively through the skin to the fat cell layer by massage has not, however, been proven.

A recently published study showed that after a daily application of an aminophyllin-containing cream over a period of five weeks, the thighs had shrunk in circumference by about 1 cm ($\frac{1}{2}$ inch). Unfortunately, however, these results cannot be treated as conclusive, since measurements alone are not very accurate.

Since other drugs can be delivered through the skin using patches, it is reasonable to expect that active ingredients, such as caffeine and vitamin E, can also be delivered effectively to the deeper layer of fat from a cream applied to the skin. Massage increases absorption by heating the skin. I recommend that you try the cream of your choice and judge for yourself.

I have researched and developed *Longévité*® Cellulite Treatment Lotion, which contains not only caffeine but also a high concentration of natural vitamin E. This vitamin E acts on connective tissue so that the septae

surrounding the fat cells do not become thicker and the surface of the skin retains its elasticity for longer.

Before you massage, apply lotion, gel or oil using a gentle sweeping motion. Then use one of three techniques:

1 The Hand/Heel Technique

Best for the thighs. Bend your wrist back, lifting the palm and fingers, then firmly massage your thigh just above the knee. Work upwards towards the upper thigh. Next massage the front and back of your thigh, starting at the knee and moving upwards. Don't forget the area just below the buttocks. Massage each thigh for at least one minute.

2 The Knuckle Technique

Best for the upper arms. Extend the arm to be massaged in front of you with the elbow bent, and make a fist with the other hand. Press

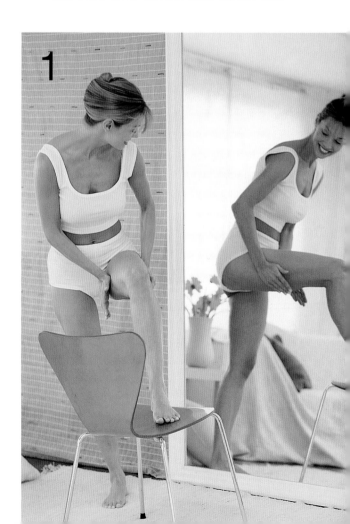

your knuckles along your upper arm, massaging firmly from the elbow to the top of the arm. Repeat at least 20 full strokes on each arm.

3 Petrissage

Best for the "love handles" of the lower back. Petrissage can also be used on the upper arms, but do not use this technique on the thighs as it may encourage the formation of tiny spider veins. Grasp the fold of skin on your lower back between your thumb and fingers, then squeeze and twist as if you were kneading dough. Massage both sides of your back simultaneously for at least one minute.

THE SUN

The sun is your skin's worst enemy! Always protect yourself from the sun. Individuals who have pale skin are at the greatest risk, but no one is immune to the dangerous effects of the sun. All sun exposure is bad; there is no such thing as a safe tan! Tanning is simply the visible evidence of the damage the sun is causing to your skin.

There is no doubt that the sun ages your skin prematurely, causing wrinkles, loss of elasticity, leathery texture and blotchy dark and sometimes rough spots (the latter may be precancerous). Even worse, the sun causes skin cancer, especially in those who have had blistering sunburns or who have moles, a previous skin cancer, or a genetic family history of skin cancer.

If you are tempted to camouflage your cellulite with a tan, get your tan from a bottle of self-tanner rather than from the sun. Be sure to apply the self-tanner carefully and evenly and to wash your hands thoroughly after applying (or the darkest tan will be on your palms).

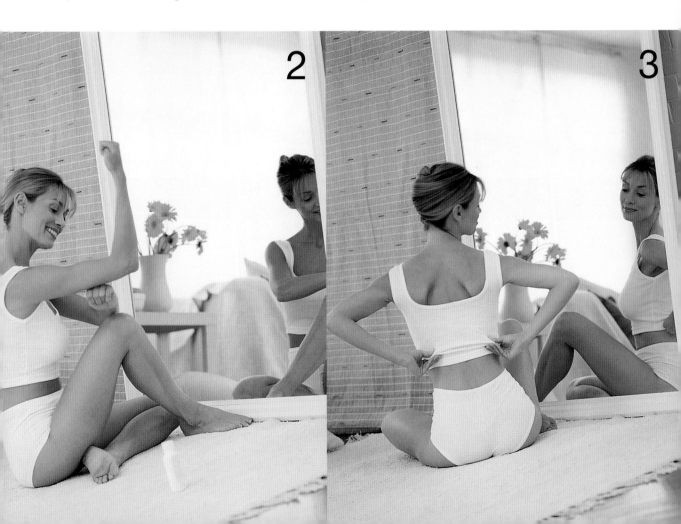

Your Positive Progress

I find it helpful to keep a diary, to "score" myself and to chart my progress. A diary inspires me to keep going. Since the *Thin Thighs* plan is done at home, without the advantage (or expense) of a rigidly scheduled spa or the supervision of a trainer, the discipline is entirely individual. Keeping a diary shows what you're really doing each day. By taking a few minutes to think about yourself, to write your thoughts, you will identify your weak points so that you can improve And you will realize how much you have accomplished!

Even if keeping a diary is not your usual custom, I would encourage you to complete the first few lines of the diary each day. Use the format of the diary shown below, which you can photocopy as many times as you need and use every day.

First, list your weight that day, taken in the morning with no clothes, just after awakening and emptying your bladder. Whether you are trying to lose weight or simply maintain your weight, it does help to weigh yourself each day. If you weigh more than the day before, you need only cut down on what you eat that day. Eating slightly smaller portions (especially at dinner) and no dessert usually does the trick. This regular monitoring allows you to maintain your weight, so that extra pounds don't slowly accumulate to the point of disaster. Some dieters, however, prefer to weigh themselves only once each week. Do what best helps you! If you are trying to lose weight, don't be discouraged if you hit a plateau when you are not measurably losing for several days. As long as you don't gain weight, you are on the right track.

Your Cellulite Reduction Diary

Week number:_____ Day:_____ Date:_____ Weight:_____

Why I am happy with myself today: _____

My Improvement Motto today:_____

Exercise

	Goal	Achievement
Pressometrics # sets		
Streamline Stretches # sets		
Twelve-Minute Miracle # sets		
Thigh Thinners time		
Aerobics time		

Diet

	Goal	Achievement
Did I follow my diet plan today at breakfast?	yes/no	
lunch?	yes/no	
dinner?	yes/no	
snacks?	yes/no	
Did I binge today?	yes/no	

Diary

Always keep your target in mind. If you are over 30, this may be your weight when you were in your early twenties. Also, remember that replacing fat with muscle can slightly increase your weight, so don't be discouraged if you have exercised and are a bit heavier.

Next, list why you are happy with yourself. Optimism and happiness can only help. Each day we can always find one special reason to be happy: the sun is shining! you feel really energetic! you did your set of the **Twelve-Minute Miracle** before your children awakened or your phone interrupted!

Think of an improvement to emphasize that day: repeat to yourself a positive phrase, an Improvement Motto, to reinforce that behaviour. "Stand tall." "Feel energy." "Breathe deep." "Walk tight." "Squeeze that fat." "Savour each bite." "Water is wonderful." By emphasizing one small good practice each day, you will quickly make it a part of your life.

Your next entry in the diary is your exercise plan for that day – the number of sets of **Pressometrics**, **Streamline Stretches**, the **Twelve-Minute Miracle**, the **Thigh Thinners** or **Aerobics**.

Finally, record how well you followed your diet plan throughout the day. Whether you did or didn't accomplish your goal, the achievement, or the guilt, will stimulate your positive action for the next day!

Weekly Achievement

Your Weekly Achievement Review (page 124-125) is quite important – just to keep track of whether you are really following your GREFLOFS diet and your exercise plan.

Of course, you may not have been perfect *every* day, but accomplishing this at least five days each week is really great! Be kind to yourself and pat yourself on the back for any accomplishments! You deserve it!

The most important bottom line is, how do you really feel about your body? Now is the time for you to evaluate yourself honestly in the privacy of your own home, being sure not to be too critical. Take the most important test of all: The Reflection Reaction. Look at yourself in the mirror to judge whether the dimply appearance of cellulite is terrible (+3), bad (+2), minimal (+1), or non-existent (0). Your goal should be simply to demonstrate to yourself that you improve. Record these observations in the Weekly Achievement Review and you will be proud of your ever-better reflection.

Next, measure your waist; hips (at the widest point); right and left upper thighs ; left and right mid thighs; and right and left low thighs (just above the knee bone). Repeat all of these measurements every four weeks and record in the Weekly Achievement Review. Although each one may change only a little and some not at all, each month you will be happy to see a loss in the sum of all measurements and even small losses will make a tremendous improvement in your silhouette! Your goal will be to lose about 2.5–5 cm (1–2 inches) altogether.

How about your weekly Reflection Reaction! Do you look better than you did the week before, with a smoother contour over your areas of cellulite?

This *Thin Thighs* Lifestyle means for you a healthier, more enjoyable life. You will feel better, you will look better, and have fun!

Weekly Achievement

	START	WK.1	WK.2	WK.3	WK.4	WK.5
Date						
Weight						
Reflection Reaction *						
Measurements (cm or inches)						
Waist						
Hip						
Upper Thigh L/R						
Mid Thigh L/R						
Low Thigh L/R						
Sum of all measurements						
Diet # days goal met						
Exercise Total # sets						
Pressometrics						
Streamline Stretches						
Twelve-Minute Miracle						
Thigh Thinners						
Aerobic hours						
Review						
Did I follow my GREFLOFS plan this week?		yes/no	yes/no	yes/no	yes/no	yes/no
Of what am I most proud in keeping on my GREFLOFS plan?						
What was my biggest problem in keeping on my GREFLOFS plan?						
Did I follow my exercise plan this week?		yes/no	yes/no	yes/no	yes/no	yes/no
What was my greatest joy in exercising?						
What was my biggest problem in exercising?						
My best improvement this week:						
My behaviour to emphasise next week:						

Review

* Grade the dimply appearance of your cellulite:
"+" if improved, "0" if the same, "-" if worse.

WK.6	WK.7	WK.8	WK.9	WK.10	WK.11	WK.12	GOAL
yes/no	yes/no	yes/no	yes/no	yes/no	yes/no	yes/no	yes/no
yes/no	yes/no	yes/no	yes/no	yes/no	yes/no	yes/no	yes/no

Index

Publisher's Acknowledgments

Bodysuits kindly supplied by 'Sportique Fitness' UK.
For catalogue of the full range of fitness wear, phone 01773 608880.

Dishes kindly provided by Waterford Wedgwood and Rosenthal.
For catalogue and the full range of tableware, visit 158 Regent Street,
London W1R 5TA, or phone 020 7734 7262, fax 020 7287 1238

Thanks to Carol Bateman BASRD for nutritional analysis on the recipes
and to Barbara Horn for the metric and imperial conversions

Longévité® Skin Care and Cellulite Treatment Products

Researched and formulated by Dr Karen Burke, Longévité® Skin Care and Cellulite Treatment products are now available. For information on the exclusive Longévité® line, please write to:

Longévité®, c/o Cambertown Ltd, Goldthorpe, Rotherham, South Yorkshire, S63 7BL, United Kingdom. Or telephone or fax Longévité® c/o Cambertown Telephone: 01709 890666 Fax: 01709 897787

If you leave your name and mailing address, we will be pleased to mail you at no cost or obligation a descriptive leaflet and order form.